Why It's Hard To

QUIT SUGAR

JANE NEISH

Alfred Media

This book is for John who made my dreams come true.

For my father who waited a long time to see it.
And for my mother and aunt who couldn't wait long enough.

I love you all.

Contents

Introduction.......................................9

Why We Are Surrounded By Sugar...............19

Why We Love Sugar.........................45

Why We Get Cravings For Sugar....................71

Why We Lose Control Of Our Sugar

Consumption.................................103

Why Sugar Is Hard To Quit.........................135

Suggested Reading...............................163

Acknowledgements.................................165

Introduction

If you can't control your sugar consumption, however hard you try, this book is for you. Many of us consume more sugar than we want to because we develop cravings for it that are hard to ignore. I know because I was one of those people. I spent most of my life battling my cravings before I finally found the escape route.

I eventually stumbled across the secret that turned me from someone who couldn't resist sugar into someone who can eat a square of chocolate and put the rest away. And it wasn't hard to do. I discovered that the reason we get stuck in a lifelong battle with our cravings is that we try to control them, instead of switching them off. We do the opposite of what we need to do and this book explains why we do this. If you find it impossible to imagine that you can lose your 'Sweet Tooth', believe me, I know how you feel. I was born with a whole mouthful of them.

My Struggle With Sugar

I had a problem with sugar before I even knew what sugar was. In my baby photos, I look like a seal pup. I was 'the fat kid' in school in the days before childhood obesity. (There were only two of us in the whole school who were struggling with our weight).

As a teenager, I slimmed down but my battle with my cravings continued. I would feel weak-willed when I gave in and deprived of my treats when I didn't. I could never keep sweet foods in the house because I would trail endlessly backwards and forwards to get 'just a little bit' until they were gone.

I tried to get back in control over and over again. I regularly quit sugar and I tried every new diet in the hope that it would set me free – with varying success.

Sometimes I couldn't even make it through a day without sugar. I would lie in bed at night, vowing that I would never touch it again, and still eat my way through a multi-pack of chocolate bars the next morning.

Occasionally I'd manage to stay off sugar for long enough to get rid of my cravings. But it would always creep back into my diet again because I still felt a nagging desire to consume it whenever it crossed my path. I knew from bitter experience that even one mouthful would be the start of a slippery slope that would lead to more - and would eventually result in the return of my cravings.

However, after battling with my cravings, literally for

decades, I finally discovered how to free myself from them. It was a long time to spend on something that turned out to be quite easy in the end.

Free At Last

I finally managed to escape my cravings several years ago and my life today is a world away from my old sugar-filled one. My sleep has improved, along with my mood, my energy levels, my ability to concentrate and my appearance. It's not an exaggeration to say that my life has improved enormously in ways that I couldn't have predicted.

Sugar rarely makes an appearance in my diet now which seems funny given the amount of space that it used to take up in my head. Now, I consume sugar only when I really want to and not just because I can't resist it.

I can eat in restaurants without spending the entire meal thinking about the dessert menu. I can be surrounded by thousands of sweet foods in a supermarket without having to battle to resist them. And I can buy boxes of chocolates as gifts without worrying that I will eat them before I get the chance to pass them on. I no longer bother with sugar substitutes because I'm no longer scared to have a sweet treat occasionally. I know that I won't lose control of it like I did so often in the past.

11

More importantly, I don't have to make any effort to control the amount of sugar in my diet now. No one is more surprised at this than I am because I have absolutely no willpower around sugar. I never have and I never will.

After years of trying to resist my cravings, I discovered that my lack of willpower wasn't the problem. In fact, it is simply impossible to use your willpower to control your cravings. To take control of your sugar consumption you need to look at sugar in an entirely new way.

*

Why Sugar Is Hard To Quit

If you are struggling to resist sugar, it isn't because you are not trying hard enough. It's because you are falling into one of the traps that will stop you from succeeding however hard you try. I call these traps Willpower, Withdrawal and Want.

The Willpower Trap

We instinctively try to get back in control by using willpower to resist our cravings. But if you've ever tried to do this you'll know that your willpower can suddenly disappear –

usually at the time that you need it the most. You vow to quit, you are determined to succeed but somehow you just can't do it. This doesn't happen because you are weak-willed. It happens because your sugar cravings can switch your willpower off.

Often our willpower evaporates straight away and we find ourselves consuming sugar again within a few hours of quitting. But sometimes we get lucky and we manage to resist a little longer. When this happens we think that we are on the right track but we are actually heading for the second trap, 'Withdrawal'.

The Withdrawal Trap

Withdrawal is the 'reward' we get when we successfully resist our cravings. It's that unpleasant period that makes us feel every kind of miserable. We try to stick it out in the hope that we are on the way to getting rid of our cravings but we find that our cravings increase and our willpower drops even lower.

A lack of willpower and the misery of withdrawal end most of our attempts to quit. But occasionally, if we try really hard and we get really lucky, we make it through Withdrawal and our cravings disappear. When this happens, we think that we have succeeded, but we often fall straight into the final trap – 'Want'.

The Want Trap

We don't usually escape our cravings for long because, once they've gone, we discover that we still want to consume sugar. In fact, we begin to feel deprived without it.

We can't imagine not eating any for the rest of our life. How can we turn down wedding cake or be the only one in the restaurant to refuse pudding? We decide to return to sugar but we promise ourselves that this time we won't let it get out of control.

However, despite our best attempts, it's not long before our occasional treat becomes a regular treat and our regular treat becomes a daily treat. Our cravings return and we begin battling them all over again. We get locked into a cycle where we are either struggling to quit sugar or struggling to stay off it.

Sugar becomes both our torment and our treat and controlling it becomes a lifelong battle. We feel bad when we have cravings because we don't like to feel out of control. We feel bad when we are quitting because we suffer the misery of Withdrawal. And we feel bad when we succeed because we miss our treats.

We want to get rid of our cravings and keep our treats but we end up being deprived of our treats and locked in a constant battle to avoid the return of our cravings. Fortunately, there is an easier way.

The Easy Way To Quit Sugar

Sugar is hard to quit because, from the very first mouthful, our brain begins to track it. That's why it calls to us from inside the cupboard. The traps that stop us from quitting are created by our **brain**. Quite simply, we make our brain dependent on sugar so once we try to take it away, it's not happy.

When we reduce our sugar consumption, we plunge into Withdrawal because we are removing the sugar that our brain now needs so it switches off our willpower to force us back to it. If we battle hard we can sometimes fight off our brain's demands for sugar for a short time but certainly not for the rest of our life.

Even if we get through Withdrawal we usually return to sugar because, although our brain no longer needs sugar, it still wants us to consume it. It's hard to resist sugar for a short time but it's simply impossible to resist it forever. And the final irony is that, because of the way that sugar affects our brain, we are always convinced that we will succeed the next time we try to quit so we keep trying - even though we fail over and over again.

You don't need to wage war on sugar. You don't need to battle your cravings and you don't need to give up your treats because sugar is not the problem. If it was, we would all experience cravings for it – but we don't.

It's your uncontrollable desire to consume it that is the problem. You crave sugar because your brain is telling you to consume it. The ways that we instinctively try to get back in control don't work because they focus on removing sugar from our diet instead of removing sugar from our brain.

To get back in control, you need to switch off your brain's need for sugar, instead of trying to switch off the supply of sugar that your brain needs. When you remove your brain's need for sugar you can avoid the traps that stop you from succeeding.

- You don't need to use Willpower to resist your cravings if you switch them off.
- You don't plunge into Withdrawal if your brain no longer needs sugar.
- And you don't constantly Want to consume it if you have removed your brain's ability to track it.

It's easy to control the amount of sugar that you eat when your brain isn't constantly telling you to consume it. But you will be trying (and failing) to control your cravings forever if you don't remove the cause of them.

*

How This Book Will Help You

Switching your cravings off is much easier than trying to control them. But few of us discover this secret because, although it is easy to do, it is not easy to see. We try to control our cravings instead of removing them because we aren't aware of the changes that sugar makes to our brain.

I hope that this book will save you years of frustration by explaining how sugar changes your brain and triggers your cravings. Once you understand how these changes are keeping you hooked, it becomes easy to see why you are finding it so hard to take control. We'll begin by looking at why we love sugar and how it creates the cravings that keep us hooked.

In Chapter 1 we look at what sugar actually is, find out how it affects our body and discover the reason that it has exploded into our diet in recent decades. In Chapter 2 we'll find out how it changes our brain to create our desire for more.

In Chapter 3 we'll discover how sugar creates our cravings and find out why they are so hard to resist. In Chapter 4 we'll look at how our cravings drive our sugar consumption higher and higher - without us even noticing - by changing our diet and our eating patterns. And in Chapter 5 we'll look at why quitting, cutting back or using a sugar substitute can make our cravings worse and we'll find out why we keep trying to make these 'solutions' work, despite our lack of success.

Once you really understand the problem you can take action to regain control and the second book in this series 'The Easy Way To Quit Sugar' will show you how to do this. You'll find more details at the end of this book.

Finally, I've also created a free guide - 'How To Measure The Effects Of Sugar On Your Body' - which outlines easy, low-cost ways to measure the impact of your sugar consumption. Measuring the effects of sugar can help you in two ways. It can strengthen your determination to get back in control and it can provide you with a way to track your progress once you begin to take action.

You can download a copy at the following address:-

http://www.janeneish.com/measure/

Let's begin by finding out how we got into this mess.

1

Why We Are Surrounded By Sugar

Sugar is everywhere. It's in our shops, our schools, our workplaces and even our hospitals. We eat it when we are celebrating and it cheers us up when we are sad. We love sugar because we evolved to seek out sweet food. But we struggle to control the amount that we eat because we have created sugars that are so concentrated that they overwhelm our body and brain.

It is the mismatch between the sugars that our ancestors ate and the sugars that we have created that causes us problems. We are living in a world full of concentrated sugars with a body that evolved to survive in a world where sugar was hard to find. When it comes to sugar, we really have created too much of a good thing.

In this chapter, we'll find out what sugar actually is, find out how it came to be in so many of our foods and discover why it is just too concentrated for us.

What Sugar Actually Is

Processed sugar is a very recent addition to our diet but we have been eating natural sugars for millions of years. Sugars, which are also known as 'saccharides', are found in plants.

Plants get the energy that they need by using sunlight to create sugars using a process called 'photosynthesis' – so sugar is a type of fuel.

Energy From The Sun → Fuel For Plants (Stored As Sugar)

We can't get energy directly from sunlight but we can use the sugars that the plants have made. We call foods that provide us with fuel in the form of sugar 'carbohydrates'. If we consume more sugar than we need to fuel our daily activities, we can store the extra sugar for later use by converting it into fat.

Energy From The Sun → Fuel For Plants (Stored As Sugar) → Fuel For Us (Stored As Fat)

Plant-eating animals (herbivores) also use sugars for fuel and they also store extra sugar as fat. And animals that prey on other animals (carnivores) can use the fat that has been stored by their prey as fuel and they also store extra fuel as fat. This is the 'Food Chain' – energy from the sun is converted into fuel (sugar) by plants and this fuel can then be passed between animals and humans as fat.

Energy From The Sun → Fuel For Plants (Sugar) → Fuel For Animals (Fat) → Fuel For Us (Fat)

We are omnivores. This means that we can use both sugar and fat as fuels. We can also use protein, which is used to build cells in both plants and animals, as a fuel. But we usually only burn it for fuel if we can't find enough sugar or fat to eat.

We measure the amount of fuel that we get from our food in calories or kilojoules. Because plants store fuel as sugar, virtually all the calories that we get from plants – from our vegetables, beans, grains, roots, tubers and fruits - come from sugars, with a small amount from the protein that they are made from. (With the exception of the few plants that create fruits that contain fat instead of sugar - nuts, coconut, olives, avocado). And because animals store fuel as fat, virtually all the calories that we get from animal foods come from fat, with a small amount from the protein that they are made from. (The exception being milk which contains both sugar and fat).

So when we eat vegetables we are consuming sugar - even when we are consuming the ones that don't taste sweet, like broccoli or Brussels sprouts. We associate sugar with a sweet taste but most of the sugars that plants create are made from building blocks of a sugar called 'glucose' which isn't very sweet. Even foods that contain large amounts of glucose (such as potatoes or grains) don't taste sweet to us. These foods contain sugars that are made from long chains of glucose that we call 'starch' so we refer to these foods as 'starchy carbohydrates'.

The sweet taste that we associate with sugar comes from another type of sugar called 'fructose'. Fructose is about twice as sweet as glucose. It is much rarer and is always found along with glucose, never on its own. As its name suggests, it is mostly found in fruit which is why fruits generally taste sweeter than vegetables.

Glucose and fructose are 'monosaccharides' which means 'single sugars'. These are the smallest units of sugar that exist and all the sugars that are found in plants are created from different combinations of these two building blocks. (Lactose, the sugar that is found in milk, is made from glucose and another monosaccharide called 'galactose'). The stuff that we know as processed sugar is a type of sugar called 'sucrose' that we extract from sugar cane and sugar beet. Sucrose is a unit of fructose joined to a unit of glucose – so it is known as a 'disaccharide' which means 'two sugars'. So now we know what sugar is (a fuel) and where it is found (in plants), let's look at why we find it so attractive.

Why We Are Attracted To Sugar

Today, we are surrounded by foods that are full of sugar (and fat) so we have no problems finding the fuel that we need to survive but things were very different for our hunter-gatherer ancestors. They lived in a world where fuel was hard to come by and hunger would have been a constant threat.

Our ancestors faced two big challenges in their search for sugar:- the supply of sugar varied dramatically at different times of the year and much of it was locked inside plants that were inedible.

The Supply Of Sugar Was Variable

We have access to sugar all year round but this wasn't the case for our hunter-gatherer ancestors because all of their sugar came from foraging for plants. This meant that sugar was easier to find in spring and summer, when the plants were growing and reproducing, than in autumn and winter when the plants became dormant.

The best sources of sugar were only available for a very limited time because sugar is most concentrated in the parts of the plant that are used for reproduction so that the new plant has the fuel that it needs to grow until it has enough leaves to be able to create its own fuel from sunlight.[1] Sugar is concentrated in grains and beans (which are the seeds of a new plant), fruits (which are the containers for seeds) and tubers, such as potatoes (which are a way for the plant to store fuel underground to create a new plant the following year).

In fact, many of the 'vegetables' that we eat today – such as aubergines, peppers, cucumbers, tomatoes, courgettes – are actually fruits. (Anything that contains a seed is a fruit). We forget that they are seasonal because we have year round access to them. For most of the year, the bulk of our ancestors' diet would have consisted of leaves,

---

1   Gundry, Steven R. Dr. Gundry's *Diet Evolution*. 1st ed. New York: Crown Publishers, 2008. p37

roots and shoots - the parts of a plant that contain only small amounts of sugar.

The Sugar Was Hard To Access

Our ancestors couldn't even eat some the most concentrated sources of sugar when they were available. Plants don't want their grains, beans or tubers to be eaten because these are the 'seeds' that will create future plants. They make them hard to eat – either by covering them with a protective outer layer (which we can't digest) or by filling them with bitter-tasting toxins. We eat these foods today because it is easy for us to remove the inedible parts and to cook the rest but it is thought that our hunter-gatherer ancestors only ate these foods if they were starving.

The leafy greens that made up most of our ancestors' diet were low in sugar and high in fibre. Fibre is the stuff that makes plants rigid. It creates the 'bones' of the plant - so leaves and stems contain a lot of it. Unfortunately, we can't use fibre as a fuel because we can't digest it. It fills us up and reduces the amount that we can eat. This was not good news for our ancestors who were often struggling to find enough fuel to survive. They had no domesticated animals so they didn't have access to the sugar that is found in milk and although they could hunt for animals to get fuel from fat, animals at the bottom of the food chain need to eat plants to be able to create fat – so when sugar was in short supply, fat was too.

We evolved in a world where fuel was very hard to find so the ability to find sugar (and fat) and the motivation to do so was crucial to our survival. This means that we evolved to be highly attracted to foods that are high in sugar and fat. We even love the glucose-based sugars that are not very sweet which is why we use high sugar foods like bread and potatoes as 'comfort foods', rather than low sugar ones, such as lettuce and chard. But the sugar that we are most attracted to is the one that tastes sweet – fructose. We are highly motivated to seek it out. Our drive to find and consume fructose may have developed in response to fruit.

Fruit would have been a very important part of our ancestors' diet because it would have been the only concentrated source of sugar that was easy to access. Plants use barriers and toxins to try to stop themselves and their seeds from being eaten but they make fruit easy to eat because they **want** their fruit to be eaten. Fruit seeds are not harmed when they are carried through the digestive system of a bird, animal or human so when fruit is eaten, the seeds can be spread over a wide area. This helps the plants to survive because if the plants in one area are killed, by drought or flood for example, the plants in another area may survive.

Plants evolved sweet fruit because the more attractive

it was to eat, the more seeds they could spread. And we evolved to find fruit attractive because it was a valuable source of fuel. The sweeter the taste, the more attractive we find it and the more we can eat. This love of sugar that we have inherited from our ancestors has been the driving force behind the explosion of sugar in our diet. Our foods are full of sugar today because these are the foods that we are motivated to eat.

How Sugar Crept Into Our Diet

About 10,000 years ago our ancestors began to replace gathering and hunting with farming. Farming increased our ancestors' chances of survival because it enabled them to add two new sources of sugar to their diet – milk (from domesticated animals) and grains[2]. Earlier generations were unable to consume grain because it has a protective (and inedible) outer layer made of fibre. When our ancestors found a way to remove this outer layer and began to grow grains for food they were able to dramatically increase their sugar supply.

Grains had two advantages over greens. They were easy to store so our ancestors had access to sugar during the autumn and winter when plants were no longer growing

2   Ibid, p27

and fruiting. And they contained more sugar than greens because they contained fuel for a new seedling. By removing the fibre from the outside of the grain, our ancestors were able to eat the high sugar centre. The porridges and bread that they created were the first high sugar foods.

This leap in food processing was the beginning of the high sugar diet that we have today because when our ancestors removed the fibre from grain they created a whole new type of carbohydrate – the 'refined carbohydrate'. Refined carbohydrates are just plant foods, like grains, that have had their fibre removed.

By removing the fibre from grains, our ancestors didn't just create foods that helped them to survive the winter, they created foods that they really liked to eat because removing the fibre from a plant makes the sugar more concentrated. And the more concentrated the sugar, the more we like it. We are surrounded by high sugar foods today because the evolution of our food has been driven by our desire to create foods that contain more of the sugar that we love and less fibre that we don't - and we have become better and better at it.

Nowadays, we no longer need to rely on refined carbohydrates to survive the winter because advances in farming and transportation mean that most of us have year-round access to fruit and vegetables. But the proportion of refined carbohydrates in our diet has grown and grown. We are surrounded by a dizzying number of these high sugar foods because these are the foods that we love to eat. In fact, if you removed all the refined carbohydrates from a supermarket most of the foods on display – the bread, cakes, crackers and biscuits, rice cakes, juices and drinks, cereals and pasta, rice and noodles, sweets, chocolate, sauces, soups and ready meals - would disappear.

Of course, the refined carbohydrate that we find most attractive is processed sugar. We love sugar because it is a concentrated source of both glucose and the fruit sugar that we love most, fructose. The sweetest fruits are around 30% fructose and most are much lower (some as low as 4%) but sugar is 50% fructose. Sugar has given us year round access to fructose and enabled it to make the jump out of fruit and into the rest of our food.

Our hunter-gatherer ancestors would have loved the cakes and sweets that we eat today as much as we do but sugar has become a large part of our diet only recently and this has happened because globalisation has made sugar cheap. Go back a couple of generations and sugar was so expensive that it was literally locked away. We were more likely to use it to make an ornament for the dining table to impress our friends than to eat it for dessert.

It dominates our diet today because it is loved by food manufacturers and consumers alike. Manufacturers love it because it's cheap, has a long shelf life and is easy to process so it can be added to a wide range of foods. And we prefer to buy the foods – both savoury and sweet – that contain it.

We have moved from the low sugar/high fibre diet of our ancestors to a diet that is completely opposite. The scale of this change is incredible. It has been estimated that our ancestors consumed about 100g of fibre per day[3] and about 22 teaspoons of sugar **over a year** – about the same amount as two soft drinks contain nowadays.[4] In comparison, the average American consumes around 12g of fibre (around 90% less than our ancestors)[5] and 22 teaspoons of sugar **per day**.[6] We have access to more sugar, in more concentrated forms, than at any time in history. There is probably more of it in your kitchen right now than your ancestors ate over their entire lifetime.[7]

By increasing our sugar supply, we solved our hunger problem (in the rich parts of the world at least) and, as a bonus, we created foods that we love to eat. But the news is not all good because removing the fibre from our foods created fuels that are too concentrated for us to use.

3   Leach J. D. "Evolutionary Perspective on Dietary Intake and Colorectal Cancer," Eur. J. Clin. Nutr. 61 (2007): 140-42 cited in Lustig, Fat Chance 1st ed. London: Fourth Estate, 2013, p131

4   Johnson R K et al., "Dietary Sugars Intake and Cardiovascular Health: A Scientific Statement from the American Heart Association." Circulation 120 (2009): 1011-20 cited in Lustig, *Fat Chance*, p118

5   Leach "Evolutionary Perspective' cited in Lustig, Robert H. Fat Chance, p131

6   Johnson, "Dietary Sugars cited Lustig. *Fat Chance*, p118

7   De Vany, Arthur. The De Vany Diet. 1st ed. London: Vermilion, 2012.

The reason that sugar has been linked to many health problems is that there is a mismatch between the sugars that we evolved to eat and the sugars that we want to eat. This mismatch is also the reason that we find it hard to control the amount of sugar in our diet.

To find out why let's look at what happens to sugar when we eat it.

How We Process Sugar

The processed sugar that we consume today is made of the same sugars – glucose and fructose - that we have been consuming for millions of years. When we consume any kind of sugar, whether it's from a cookie or a carrot, the sugar is broken down into single units of glucose and fructose and these are then processed by different pathways in our body. However, the effect that they have on us is very different when the sugar has been removed from the plant that made it.

How We Process Glucose

When we eat a food that contains glucose, the glucose is absorbed from our small intestine into our bloodstream. We always have some glucose in our bloodstream which we use to power our cells. The measurement of how much glucose we have in our bloodstream is called our 'blood sugar level'. When our blood sugar level begins to rise, a large gland that lies behind our stomach called our 'pancreas' releases a hormone called 'insulin' into our bloodstream.

Insulin is like a key that fits into receptors on the outside of our cells. It unlocks the door to the cell so that the glucose can go inside where it can be burned to provide us with energy. The more glucose we have in our bloodstream, the more insulin we need to release to move the glucose into our cells. About 80% of the glucose that we consume is processed by our cells in this way and the remaining 20% is processed by our liver.

Any glucose that is isn't used by our cells immediately is put into storage – either as a type of quick-release fuel called 'glycogen' or as fat. We don't store much glucose as glycogen (it makes up about 1-2% of our muscles and around 8% of our liver) because glycogen provides an emergency store of water as well as fuel which makes it heavy and bulky.[8]

When we consume glucose from a natural source, like a carrot, the glucose reaches our bloodstream slowly because our digestive enzymes have to work hard to separate the sugar from the fibre but when we consume processed sugar

[8]   Gundry, *Diet Evolution*, p74

the glucose can move into our bloodstream much more rapidly because the fibre has already been removed. The less fibre a food contains, the faster the glucose is able to travel and the greater the rise in our blood sugar.

'Highly refined carbohydrates' like white bread and white rice create a greater surge in our blood sugar than wholemeal bread and brown rice because more of the fibre has been removed. Even blending fruit and vegetables to make a smoothie increases the speed that the glucose reaches our bloodstream because we can digest the fibre more easily once it has been broken down.

These surges in our blood sugar are not normal. They were almost impossible for our ancestors to experience because they didn't remove the fibre from their foods but we eat so many refined carbohydrates that can create them many times a day. We have even created scales to measure the impact that the glucose from refined carbohydrates has on our bloodstream - the 'glycemic load' (GL) which measures how much glucose a food contains and 'the glycemic index' (GI) which measures the speed that it reaches our bloodstream.

Unrefined carbohydrates are at the bottom of the glycemic index because they contain small amounts of glucose and large amounts of fibre (the only exceptions being dates and potatoes). Grains (and especially flour) are at the top because grains are concentrated sources of glucose and we have to break down or remove most of the fibre just to make them edible.

Two slices of bread or a single bagel contain about 6 teaspoons of this sugar – which is around six times more than the amount that we should have in our bloodstream.[9]

Refined sugar appears lower on the glycemic index than refined grain because only 50% of it is glucose – so adding sugar to a bowl of cereal actually lowers the glucose surge that it creates in our bloodstream.

*

Surges in our blood sugar are a problem because glucose can damage our cells. It can bind to proteins and change their shape so that they cannot be used to build or repair tissues – a process which is known as 'glycation'.[10]

Glycation creates 'Advanced Glycation End Products' (suitably called AGES) which accumulate over our lifetime and create inflammation and ageing – they create wrinkles in our skin and in our organs.[11]

---

9   Gedgaudas, Nora T. *Primal Body, Primal Mind.* 1st ed. Rochester, Vt.: Healing Arts Press, 2011

10   Lustig, *Fat Chance*, p121

11   Gedgaudas, *Primal Body*, p126

We evolved to use glucose as a fuel so we evolved a way to prevent this damage by releasing antioxidants from a part of our cell called the 'peroxisome'. But the problem is that the more glucose our cells are processing, the more antioxidants we need to produce and, if we can't produce enough of them, our cells become damaged and may even die. Plants are packed with the antioxidants that we need but, when we remove the fibre from them to create refined carbohydrates we also remove the antioxidants - so the more antioxidants we need, the less we get.

We have not evolved a way to reverse the damage to our cells that is caused by glycation because we didn't evolve eating foods that created surges in our blood sugar.[12] And high levels of glucose can also damage our kidneys because our body also tries to get rid of the excess by excreting it in our urine.

To stop a surge of glucose from damaging our cells, our pancreas releases a surge of insulin in response so that the glucose is moved out of our bloodstream and into our cells as quickly as possible. Unfortunately surges of insulin are also harmful because insulin is an inflammatory hormone that tells our cells to divide. We want high levels of insulin at puberty and during pregnancy (when we need our cells to divide so that we grow) but not at other times because

---

12   Borysenko, Joan. *The Plantplus Diet Solution.* 1st ed, p16

this increases our risk of cancer.[13] A high level of insulin can also create high blood pressure because the cells that surround our blood vessels grow, tightening the walls of our arteries.

As we get older, it becomes harder and harder to control surges in our blood sugar because, between the ages of 40 and 60, we lose around one-third of our muscle cells so we have fewer cells available to burn off the excess glucose.

Glucose is a natural fuel that we have always used but more concentrated sources of it are not better sources of fuel. Think of it like this – your television runs on electricity but if there is a surge in the power supply, it doesn't improve the picture, it simply damages the television because it is more than the circuits can handle. It's the same for us with glucose. It is not insulin's 'job' to correct surges in our blood sugar. We are not supposed to have these surges in our blood sugar. Now let's take a look at fructose because we process this sugar in an entirely different way.

*

13   Shaw R. J.et al., "Decoding Key Nodes in the Metabolism of Cancer Cells: Sugar and Spice and All Things Nice", F1000 Biol. Rep. 4 (2012):2 cited in Lustig, *Fat Chance* p124

How We Process Fructose

All of our cells can use glucose as a fuel but this is not true of fructose because it was never a large part of our diet. In fact, only a very small number of cells - sperm cells, some stomach cells and sometimes our kidney - can use (tiny amounts) of fructose. So virtually all the fructose that reaches our bloodstream goes to our liver to be processed.

It is actually quite hard for the fructose from fruit to reach our bloodstream. Much of it remains trapped in our gut and is used as a fuel by the bacteria that live there. But the fructose from refined sugar finds it easier to escape because the more glucose a food contains, the easier it is for fructose to cross into our bloodstream. Since sugar is 50% glucose, the fructose that it contains can cross into our bloodstream quite easily. The fructose travels around our bloodstream until it reaches our liver where it is turned into fat so, despite the claims on labels, sugar isn't really 'fat-free'.

Fructose is 'Future Fuel'. We can break down the fat that it is created by fructose to use as fuel in the future but most fructose isn't used as fuel when we eat it because few of our cells can actually use it. This wasn't a problem for our ancestors because they only ate tiny amounts of fructose but it is a problem for us because we eat large amounts of it. Large amounts of fructose become large amounts of fat and if our liver fills up with it, it can't work properly.

Large amounts of fat in our liver can lead to 'non-alcoholic fatty liver disease' (NAFLD).[14] (Fructose and alcohol are processed by our liver in the same way. The only difference between them is that alcohol is processed by our brain but fructose isn't so it doesn't make us drunk). A recent survey found that nearly one-third of the US population has NAFLD, a condition which has few or no symptoms. This makes it the most common disease in the US – an amazing statistic since the condition was only recognised as recently as the 1980s. NAFLD can progress to cirrhosis where normal liver tissue is replaced by scar tissue so our liver tries to protect itself by moving the fat to other parts of our body. This increases the amount of fat in our bloodstream and has been linked to an increased risk of heart disease and stroke. And when this fat is moved into our fat cells, it is our visceral fat cells that fill up first.[15]

Visceral fat is the 'bad' fat that we are warned about because it creates inflammation throughout our body. It's is a type of quick-release energy so it is stored around our organs and stomach where our liver has easy access to it. We can store a lot of this fat without being aware of it

14   Lustig, *Fat Chance* p150
15   Ibid, p124

because it is hidden away. Even if you look slim and you have a normal Body Mass Index (BMI), you can have enough of this fat inside you to be classed as obese. This is known as being a 'TOFI' - 'Thin on the Outside, but Fat on the Inside'.[16]

Scans carried out by Dr Eric Braverman suggest that the number of 'obese' slim people may be very high - 50% of women and 20% of men.[17]

And fat isn't the only thing that can be created by a diet that is high in fructose. When our liver has to process large amounts of fructose (more than around 50 grams), it can run short of the 'ATP' (adenosine triphosphate) that it needs to process it. If this happens, uric acid is generated as a waste product when the fructose is processed.

Animals that evolved eating a high fruit diet have an enzyme called 'uricase' that breaks down uric acid but we lack this enzyme. We can excrete uric acid in our urine but the speed at which we can remove it varies from person to person so it can build up in our body. If you get a build up of uric acid crystals you may be able to feel them under the skin on the soles of your feet – they feel like tiny

16   Thomas, E. Louise et al. "The Missing Risk: MRI And MRS Phenotyping Of Abdominal Adiposity And Ectopic Fat". Obesity 20.1 (2011): 76-87. Web.cited in Lustig, *Fat Chance*, p89
17   Shah, Nirav R. and Eric R. Braverman. "Measuring Adiposity In Patients: The Utility Of Body Mass Index (BMI), Percent Body Fat, And Leptin". PLoS ONE 7.4 (2012): e33308. Web. Ibid

pieces of grit. A build up of uric acid around the joints of our big toes can cause gout and, because uric acid blocks the action of nitric oxide which relaxes our blood vessels, it has also been linked to high blood pressure.

Fructose has also been linked to digestive problems. It can create an imbalance in our gut bacteria because it feeds our 'bad' bacteria allowing them to multiply and crowd out the 'good' ones that we need for useful things like vitamin production. (It is fibre that feeds the good ones). If we consume enough fructose to feed a large population of these bacteria, they can spread into our small intestine creating SIBO (Small Intestine Bacterial Overgrowth). This can create gas and bloating because the bacteria begin to consume the fructose (they ferment it) in the wrong part of our digestive tract.

Fructose can lead to diarrhoea because it absorbs water and it may also contribute to the breakdown of the wall of our intestine which can allow bacteria and food particles to move from our gut into our bloodstream ('leaky gut'). This can create food allergies because our immune system sees these particles as invaders and attacks them. And finally, fructose can also damage the proteins in our cells when it is travelling in our bloodstream – however, fructose damages these proteins seven times faster than glucose.[18]

18 Dills W. L. "Protein Fructosylation: Fructose and the Maillard Reaction," Am. J. Clin. Nutr. 58 (1993): 779S-87S Ibid, p123

Glucose creates problems if it reaches our bloodstream faster than we can process it. Fructose creates problems if we eat too much of it. Our ancestors ate sugars that contained low levels of fructose and glucose together with high levels of fibre which slowed the digestion of the glucose. They consumed sugars that were 'Low and Slow'. By taking away the fibre we have created sugars that are 'High and Fast'. They contain high levels of fructose and fast-digesting glucose.

Natural Sugars **Low Fructose / Slow Glucose**
Refined Sugar   **High Fructose / Fast Glucose**

We have not evolved to consume refined carbohydrates and processed sugars in large quantities, over long periods of time. The health problems that surround us today - obesity, digestive problems, diabetes, dementia, stroke, cancer and heart disease have been called the 'Diseases Of Civilisation' because they begin to appear within one generation when a population begins to eat highly refined carbohydrates. This is known as 'The Rule of 20 Years'.[19]

The bad news is that it's not just the stuff in the sugar bowl that has this effect. All refined sugars overwhelm

---

19   Price, W 1997, Nutrition and Physical Degeneration, New York: Keats Publishing cited in Gundry, *Diet Evolution*, p18

our sugar processing pathways because all refined sugars are High and Fast.

The Other Refined Sugars

Sugar has had a bad press in recent years but our body processes all refined sugars in the same way. We don't hear about problems with these other sugars simply because we don't consume them in the same quantities as white sugar. But it doesn't matter whether the sugar has come from a tree (maple syrup), a flower (honey), a cactus (agave), a fruit (date sugar) a grain (High Fructose Corn Syrup) or a vegetable (sugar beet) and it doesn't matter whether the sugar is 'organic', 'natural' or 'raw'. The only thing that matters is the concentration of the fructose and availability of the glucose. Once a sugar has been separated from the plant that created it, our body struggles to process it.

Honey and maple syrup are roughly 50% glucose and 50% fructose - the same proportion that we find in white sugar. The tiny amount of nutrients that they contain won't offset the problems that are created by the high fructose content and the fast-digesting glucose. Similarly High Fructose Corn Syrup, which can be manufactured to contain up to 90% fructose, usually contains the same proportions of glucose and fructose as white sugar because it is used as a cheap sugar substitute in processed foods.

(The glucose and fructose are not joined together as they are in sucrose though which may allow the glucose to be processed even faster or for even more of the fructose to reach our bloodstream).[20] Agave syrup and fruit purées are also high fructose syrups – just not from corn - and they can also contain more fructose than processed sugar.

All refined sugars are concentrated sources of glucose and fructose and we process all of them in the same way so when we talk about sugar, we are really talking about all of them.

The good news is that refined sugars are very easy to avoid because they only appear in processed foods. They are not in our vegetables, fruit, meat, fish, eggs, herbs or spices. But keeping them out of our diet is easier said than done (I can hear you laughing) because although we may want to avoid sugar, we just can't seem to manage it - however hard we try. The problem is that sugar doesn't just overwhelm our body – it also overwhelms our brain. Natural sugars may be better for us but it is refined sugar that we want to eat.

To find out why sugar is so hard to resist we need to look at the way that sugar changes our brain to create our desire for more.

20   Le et al, "Effects of High-Fructose Corn Syrup and Sucrose on the Pharmacokinetics of Fructose and Acute Metabolic and Hemodynamic Responses in Healthy Subjects", Metabolism 61 (2012):641-51 cited in Lustig, *Fat Chance*, p119

2

Why We Love Sugar

We think that we love sugar just because it tastes nice and that the desire to eat it simply pops into our head from time to time but this is not the case. We don't love sugar because of the way that it tastes, we love it because it makes changes to our brain that drive us to seek it out. In this chapter, we'll look at how, from the very first taste, sugar changes our brain to create our desire for more.

How Sugar Affects Our Brain

Our brain is made up of cells called 'neurons'. These cells don't actually touch but they can communicate with one another by releasing chemicals called 'neurotransmitters'.

When a neurotransmitter is released by a neuron, it can be captured by receptors on the surface of other neurons and this passes on a message. We have many different neurotransmitters that transmit many different messages.

One of them, serotonin, increases in our brain when we consume a food that contains glucose. Serotonin has many important functions. It helps to control sexual desire, appetite, sleep, memory, learning and body temperature. But we hear about it most in connection with our mood because it is serotonin that makes us feel happy.

Serotonin is created from an amino acid called 'tryptophan'. Amino acids are the building blocks of proteins and we get them from the proteins in our food. When we consume a food that contains tryptophan, the tryptophan moves into our bloodstream and from here it can cross into our brain where it can be converted into serotonin. However, tryptophan has to compete for access to our brain with all the other amino acids that are circulating in our bloodstream and many of them can cross into our brain more easily.

When we consume glucose, the insulin that is released into our bloodstream to move the glucose into our cells also removes these competing amino acids and this allows more tryptophan to cross into our brain - so when we eat a food that contains glucose we feel good.

We Consume Glucose → Our Blood Sugar Rises → Insulin Is Released → The Competing Amino Acids Are Removed → More Tryptophan Crosses Into Our Brain → Serotonin Rises

The more concentrated the glucose, the better we feel because the more insulin we release, the less competition tryptophan has. This is the reason that refined sugars make us feel happier than natural ones. When we consume refined sugar so many of the competing amino acids are removed that tryptophan can flood into our brain. A surge of glucose creates a surge of serotonin that noticeably lifts our mood for about two hours.[21]

We Consume Fast-Digesting Glucose → Our Blood Sugar Surges → We Release A Surge Of Insulin → More Of The Competing Amino Acids Are Removed → Tryptophan Floods Into Brain → Serotonin Surges

And serotonin is not the only feel-good chemical that surges in our brain when we consume sugar, two others - 'beta-endorphin' and 'dopamine' are also increased.

---

21   For more about serotonin synthesis see Kharrazian, Datis. *Why Isn't My Brain Working?.* 1st ed, p72

Sugar creates a surge of beta-endorphin that lasts for around thirty minutes. Endorphins are painkillers and beta-endorphin is one of the most powerful. It's also released during exercise and is responsible for producing the euphoria that we call the 'runners' high'. The amount of beta-endorphin that we have in our brain determines our ability to cope with pain – the higher the level, the higher our pain threshold. Babies who are given sugar become less distressed by circumcision – so you can see just how powerful this painkiller can be.[22]

And it is not just physical pain that is reduced. Beta-endorphin also lessens emotional pain and produces a sense of well-being. It makes us feel optimistic and 'on top of the world', lowers anxiety and boosts our self-esteem. When our levels of beta-endorphin are high, we feel more talkative, confident and funny. It increases our sense of connection to others and reduces feelings of isolation. (This effect that can be seen in many species – for example, young chicks that are given sugar cry less when they are removed from their mother).

And finally, a neurotransmitter called dopamine is also increased. Dopamine creates the feelings of pleasure that we get when we consume sugar and it also gives us a sense of clarity and energy.

These chemicals have an immediate and powerful effect

22   Lustig, *Fat Chance*, p61

on us. We feel energised, focused, confident, optimistic and happy. We love sugar, not because of its nice taste, but because it produces a mild euphoria.

Some of us experience a greater sense of happiness than others when we consume sugar and other refined carbohydrates because we have a larger number of receptors for these neurotransmitters. If you are someone who naturally produces a low level of a neurotransmitter, your brain evens things out by creating more receptors for it so that your neurotransmitters have a better chance of finding a receptor and delivering their message. If this is the case, the surge in your neurotransmitters that is created by refined sugar can hit a large number of receptors and deliver a very powerful message - so sugar makes you feel very good indeed.

On the other hand, if you naturally produce large amounts of a neurotransmitter, your brain reduces the number of receptors that you have for it so that the message that it creates isn't overwhelming. If this is the case, sugar makes you feel good but the effect is not as powerful. Some of us love sugar more that others simply because the neurotransmitters that are released in response to it have a more powerful effect on our brain. But it is not just a happy coincidence that sugar makes us feel good. These neurotransmitters have a purpose. They are created to ensure that we consume more sugar.

Why Our Brain Wants Us To Consume Sugar

Sugar makes us feel good because our brain wants us to consume it. We create feel-good chemicals in our brain when we do something that is good for us. By making these actions pleasurable, our brain can guide us to repeat the actions that will help us to survive.

Similarly, behaviours that are harmful (such as touching a hot surface) make us feel bad so that we will avoid these actions in the future. The creation of feelings of pleasure or pain in response to our actions is known as the 'hedonic pathway'.[23] This pathway is the driving force that keeps us alive and it is controlled by one of the chemicals that are released when we consume sugar - dopamine.

When we consume sugar, the dopamine that is released binds to receptors in an area of our brain called the 'nucleus accumbens' (which is also known as our 'Reward Centre') to create feelings of pleasure. Our brain rewards us because consuming sugar is one of the survival behaviours that it wants us to repeat. Sugar is a fuel and we need to consume fuel to survive. In fact, the ability to find sugar is so important that we have taste buds over our entire tongue to help us to identify it. The neurotransmitters that we release when we find sugar make us feel happy and energetic because when we are able to find fuel, we

23   Ibid p50 for a description of this pathway

are able to carry out behaviours that need a good supply of it, such as reproduction.

We get a bigger reward when we consume a refined sugar than when we consume a natural one because the sugar is more concentrated. Refined sugars light up our Reward Centre. We have evolved to prefer foods with a high sugar content because these foods contain more fuel so they would have given our ancestors a better chance of survival. Our brain still motivates us to consume these foods because although our world has changed, our brain has not. It is still driving us to seek out the most concentrated sources of sugar. It is our brain's reward system that drives us away from the low sugar/high fibre diet of our ancestors to the high sugar/low fibre diet that we eat today.

Our Reward Centre not only drives us to high sugar foods, it also enables us to eat more of these foods because it is the insulin that we release in response to glucose that gives the signal to stop the release of the neurotransmitters in our brain.

But insulin isn't released in response to fructose so, when a food is high in fructose, neurotransmitters are released in our brain for longer. We are able to eat more of these foods because we don't stop eating until the reward that we are getting from them stops. Plants create fruit that is high in fructose because animals are not only attracted to it, they are able to eat a lot of it – apes, for example, binge on fruit.[24] When more fruit is eaten, more seeds are spread.

The reward that we get from sugar lasts even longer than the reward we get from fruit because sugar is 50% fructose – about 20% higher than the sweetest fruit. We are also able to consume large amounts of sugar because we have removed the fibre that fills us up. Sugar creates an intense, long-lasting reward without a feeling of fullness.

However, because we evolved in a world where sugar was hard to find, it was not enough for our brain to create a love of sugar – we also needed a way to be able to find this fuel again. So our Reward Centre doesn't just create feelings of pleasure when we consume sugar, it also activates learning so that our brain can remember the source of the sugar and can prompt us to seek it out again. We all have a 'Sugar Seeking Programme'. It is this programme that creates our desire for sugar and it starts to do this from the very first taste.

Let's look at how it works.

---

24   Knott C. D. 'Changes in Orangutan Caloric Intake, Energy Balance and Ketones In Response To Fluctuating Fruit Availability' (1998) Int. Jour. Of Primatology 19:1061-79 cited in Gundry, *Diet Evolution*, p24

Our Sugar Seeking Programme

The surge of dopamine that is created when we consume sugar doesn't just create a feeling of pleasure, it also activates our memory. It enables our brain to link the information that it is receiving from our senses - about where we are and what we are doing - with the sugar that we have found. Our brain uses this information to create triggers that will help it to identify opportunities to find sugar in the future.

Our brain begins the search for these triggers from the moment that they are created and, whenever it finds one, it prompts us to look for sugar. We create these triggers in response to things in the world around us, so let's call these 'External Triggers'.

External Triggers

External Triggers can be created from any of the information that our brain receives from our senses - the sight of a sweet food (even if it's just a photograph), a scent (such as the aroma of a baking cake) or even a sound (the rustle of a sweet wrapper is easily identified by most of us). Our brain creates these triggers automatically every time we consume a food that contains sugar and it creates stronger triggers for refined sugars because they create a bigger surge in our neurotransmitters.

So if you grab a chocolate bar whilst you are out shopping, your brain will be busy linking the design of the wrapper and the name and appearance of the shop with the opportunity to find chocolate - so that next time it spots one of these triggers it can remind you to look for more.

Shop Appearance ← Chocolate → Shop Name
↓
Wrapper

Your brain doesn't know which of the bits of information will help you to find sugar again and which will not, so it creates triggers for everything. Things that we think of as being linked to sugar become triggers - such as the wrapper of the chocolate bar or the logo of the shop. But things that seem to be completely unconnected also become triggers. For example, if you were served by a sales assistant who was wearing unusual earrings or there was a yellow van parked outside the shop when you bought the chocolate, these details will also have been recorded.

Yellow Van ← Chocolate → Earrings

And your brain doesn't just collect information about the place you were in when you found the sugar. It also remembers what you were doing and when you were doing it.[25] Once our brain has created these External Triggers it constantly monitors the information that streams in from our senses to see if it can spot any of them. So when you see an advert for the chocolate bar that you bought when you were shopping or you walk past a shop that is part of the chain, that you bought it from the idea that you might like some chocolate pops into your head because your brain prompts you to seek it out. It believes that chocolate may be close by because it has spotted something that was present when you found it in the past. Just as our ancestors would have been prompted to look for berries when they saw a particular type of leaf, for example.

Sights, sounds and smells become External Triggers for the products that we buy. Manufacturers wrap their products in colourful wrappers, retailers create distinctive displays and supermarkets have in-store bakeries which create an enticing aroma because when we come across one of the triggers that we have linked to sugar, our brain tells us to look for it.

Our brain can also trigger a search for sugar in response to our activities. For example, if you stop to buy chocolate on your way home from work, your brain may prompt you to buy chocolate when you are leaving work the

---

25　Duhigg, Charles. The Power Of Habit. 1st ed. New York: Random House, 2012 p25 following day. The search for a sweet treat can easily become part of our daily routine. Of course, when we think about sugar we don't realise that we are simply reacting to a trigger that our brain has created. If the trigger has an obvious connection to sugar – for example, if we are passing a shop that sells chocolate or we see an advert for it – we think that we are reacting to the sugar, not to the trigger that we have created for the sugar.

If the trigger has no obvious connection to sugar – for example, we see a yellow van like the one that was outside the shop when we bought chocolate last time or we see someone who is wearing similar earrings to the shop assistant who served us – the idea seems to come from nowhere. We 'Just Fancy Something Sweet'. We think that we are making a spontaneous decision to treat ourselves but, in reality, we are simply reacting to a trigger that our brain has spotted. Our sugar consumption often reduces when we are away from home because we leave many of our triggers behind.

The triggers that our brain creates don't just exist in isolation, they are linked together to form a network - like a gigantic spider's web.[26] By linking the triggers together, our brain not only remembers sources of sugar, it can also predict new ones.

---

26   Ideas trigger other ideas in a 'spreading cascade' in our brain Kahneman, Daniel. *Thinking, Fast And Slow*

How Our Brain Finds New Sources Of Sugar

As we have seen, the ability to find fuel was crucial to the survival of our ancestors so our brain doesn't just remember the sources of sugar that we have found, it also uses the triggers that it has created to try to predict where we can find more. So our brain not only tells us to look for sugar when it spots an existing trigger, it also tells us to look for sugar when it identifies something that it can link to one of these triggers. For example, if you see someone wearing a necklace that is similar to the earrings that the shop assistant was wearing when you last bought chocolate, your brain will pop the idea of chocolate into your head, in case the necklace is a sign that there is chocolate nearby.

Necklace → Earrings → Chocolate

Our brain gets better and better at finding sugar because it doesn't just create and store huge numbers of External Triggers – it also learns which ones are most likely to work.

If a trigger is activated and we consume sugar again as a result, the trigger grows stronger. For example, if you are passing the shop where you bought the chocolate, your brain will give you a nudge and say 'Hey you're passing that shop again! Go in and get more chocolate!' If you do, the connection between the shop and the chocolate becomes stronger because you will create new triggers and strengthen the existing ones. Every time a trigger is successfully activated, it grows stronger. And the stronger it becomes, the more often it is activated.

Trigger Identified → You Think Of Sugar → You Consume Sugar → Trigger Strengthens

Our brain creates a more intense prompt to tell us to search for sugar if the trigger is strong because this means that the trigger has been successful in the past so we have a good chance of finding sugar again. We create strong triggers for the foods and drinks that we consume frequently and we consume these foods frequently because we have many strong triggers for them. They become our 'favourites'.

Similarly, if a trigger is activated and we don't find sugar, the trigger becomes weaker because it hasn't been unsuccessful. For example, if you see someone who is wearing a pair of earrings that are similar to the ones that the sales assistant was wearing when you last bought chocolate, your brain may tell you to look for chocolate. But since there isn't a connection between these two things, it is much less likely that you will find chocolate nearby so the trigger grows weaker.

Trigger Identified → You Think Of Sugar → You Don't Consume Sugar → Trigger Weakens

Triggers that don't have a high chance of success weaken and disappear so that we don't use fuel looking for fuel that probably isn't there. It would have been vital to erase these triggers to stop our ancestors from wasting precious fuel by walking for miles to look for berries if they were out of season for example. By continually strengthening and weakening triggers in response to our attempts to find sugar, our brain can maintain an up-to-date map in our head.

This 'Sugar Map' not only identifies opportunities to find sugar, it also ranks our chances of success. Our Sugar Seeking Programme works tirelessly searching for triggers and updating them as it learns which ones are likely to lead to sugar and which are not so every time we enjoy a sweet treat, we are improving our brain's ability to track sugar.

Our 'Sugar Map' can become very large because we are surrounded by sugar so our brain has many opportunities to find it. The more triggers we create, the more chances our brain has to be able to spot a trigger (or something that it can link to a trigger) so the more often our brain prompts us to look for sugar. And every time we consume sugar in response to one of these prompts, we strengthen our existing triggers and create even more.

This creates a vicious circle which you may recognise – the more sugar you consume, the more sugar you want.

We Consume Sugar → We Create External Triggers → Our Brain Spots A Trigger → We Consume Sugar → We Create More External Triggers

Our Sugar Seeking Programme doesn't just point out opportunities to find sugar, it also encourages us to act on them. Once a trigger has been activated, our brain doesn't want us to ignore it so it motivates us to take action by creating desire.

How Our Brain Creates Desire

We've seen that our brain releases dopamine when we consume sugar and that this activates our Reward Centre and makes us feel good. But our brain is also able to motivate us to consume sugar by activating our Reward Centre **before** we consume the sugar. By giving us a sample of the reward that we will get when we act on the prompt from our brain, we don't just think about eating something sweet, we think about how much we would like to eat something sweet.[27]

Trigger Identified → Small Reward (We Want Sugar) → We Consume Sugar → Large Reward (We Feel Good)

And just to make sure that we get the message, our brain doesn't just make us feel good when we consume sugar, it makes us feel bad when we don't. If our brain spots a trigger and we fail to find any sugar, we feel frustrated. We don't consume sugar just because it makes us feel good, we also consume it because, if we don't, we feel bad.[28]

Trigger Identified → Small Reward (We Want Sugar) → We Don't Consume Sugar → No Reward (We Feel Bad)

So, our Sugar Seeking Programme creates our love of sugar, builds a network of triggers that alert us to all the opportunities that we have to find it and prompts us to act on them by creating desire.

---

27   Duhigg, Habits p46

28   This is called a 'Prediction Error Signal' See Lehrer, Jonah. *The Decisive Moment* for more information about how we make decisions

Sugar Seeking Programme → External Triggers → Opportunity To Find Fuel → Desire

Our ability to track sources of fuel and the desire to consume them keeps us alive. We wouldn't last long if we couldn't find food or weren't interested in eating it. The problem is that our brain is much more interested in tracking refined sugars than it is in tracking natural ones. Refined sugar is an abnormally concentrated fuel that not only creates more intense feelings of pleasure, it also creates a more intense desire to seek it out. So instead of pointing out opportunities to consume vegetables and fruit, our brain is actively looking for opportunities to consume refined carbohydrates and sugar.

Our brain tracks sugar as though our life depends on it because, when we lived in a world where sugar was hard to find, it really did depend on it. Sugar may be bad for us, but it makes us feel good and it makes us want more. There is one final factor that turns our Sugar Seeking Programme into a liability in a sugar-filled world. It isn't actually under our conscious control.

*

Our Sugar Seeking Programme Is Controlled By Our Unconscious

We are not aware of the triggers that we are creating when we consume sugar because our Sugar Seeking Programme is controlled by the unconscious part of our brain. We tend to think that our unconscious is only active when we are asleep - producing our dreams and nightmares – but, in fact, it is always active. It has been estimated that this part of our brain controls at least 40% of our daily activities and some researchers think that this can rise as high as 90%. Our conscious and unconscious are not actually separate parts of our brain, they are simply two systems that run side by side.[29]

The conscious part of our brain is used for thinking, planning, maths and decision making. It's the part of our brain that we think of as 'us'. Whereas the unconscious part monitors all the processes that are taking place inside our body and all the information that is streaming in from our senses. It can also carry out learned routines. We can use our unconscious to control quite complex behaviour, such as driving a car - which is why we can drive home without remembering any details about the journey.

If your mind can wander whilst you are doing something

---

29   See Kahneman, Daniel. *Thinking, Fast And Slow* for more information about the two systems in our brain.

- for example, if you are thinking about work as you are doing the washing up or making a mental shopping list as you walk across town - it is the unconscious part of your brain that is in control of the walking and the washing up. This frees up the conscious part of our brain so that we can think about other things. We think that we consciously control all our actions simply because we take the ability to separate our thoughts from our actions for granted.[30]

But imagine how different life would be if we really did use the conscious part of our brain to control all our activities. When we woke in the morning we would have to focus our attention on dressing and washing, instead of using the unconscious part of our brain to run through our morning routine, whilst the conscious part spends the time running through our presentation, making a mental to-do list or listening to the news.

We are not aware that our brain is creating triggers for sugar and searching for them because we don't use the conscious part of our brain to do this. We are only aware of the prompt that the unconscious part of our brain creates when it has spotted a trigger for sugar and it needs the conscious part of our brain to take action to find it.[31]

---

30 'Conscious brain is a spectator not an instigator of tasks' Lewis, David. Impulse. 1st ed.

31 'Only after our brain has made a decision do we become aware of it' Lewis,

Unconscious Brain → Search For Triggers (No Awareness) → Conscious Brain → Desire For Sugar (We Are Aware Of The Prompt To Take Action)

It may seem odd to discover that the 'spontaneous' ideas that we have to treat ourselves to 'something sweet' have been planted there by our unconscious but there are good reasons why the search for fuel is controlled by this part of our brain. The unconscious part of our brain controls the actions that we need to carry out to survive because this part of our brain is older than the conscious part. To put it simply we needed to be able to search for fuel before we needed to be able to think. And the search for fuel hasn't been moved into the conscious part of our brain because the unconscious part can do this more effectively.

Let's look at the reasons why the unconscious part of our brain is better at searching for fuel.

It Can Track More Triggers

The unconscious part of our brain can track more triggers than the conscious part and it can search through more information to find them. In comparison, the conscious part

_____

David, *Impulse*

of our brain is slow and it has a limited capacity. Although we like to think that we are aware of everything that happens in the world around us, in reality, we can only focus on a tiny fraction of the information that streams in from our senses. We miss much more than we see and it is the unconscious part of our brain that tells our conscious brain where to focus its (limited) attention.

It Can Work Continuously

The unconscious part of our brain is able to search for sugar continuously because, unlike the conscious part, it can multi-task easily. If we used the conscious part of our brain to search for sugar, we would stop searching whenever our attention was focused elsewhere. But we can't forget to do something that is controlled by our unconscious.

It Frees Up The Conscious Part Of Our Brain

Being able to use the unconscious part of our brain for routine tasks keeps the conscious part free to handle anything out of the ordinary that the unconscious part of our brain can't handle.

It Uses Less Fuel

Our brain makes up only 5% of our body mass but it uses 20 - 30% of our energy[32] – more than any other organ - and the conscious part of our brain uses the most energy of all. When we are using the unconscious part of our brain to carry out a task, the activity in our brain actually drops because the conscious part can 'switch off' whilst we carry it out. So using the unconscious part of our brain minimises the amount of fuel that we use whilst we are searching for more.

However, the drawback to using this part of our brain to search for sugar is that it makes sugar hard to resist.

Why Our Desire For Sugar Can Be Hard To Resist

As we've seen, the unconscious part of our brain actively searches for sugar and when it spots a possible opportunity to find it, it tells us to look for it. We call an action that is controlled by the unconscious part of our brain that we carry out automatically in response to a trigger, a 'habit'.[33] Any action that activates our Reward Centre can become a habit. A habit is simply a pathway in our brain that locks

32   Gedgaudas, Primal Body, p230
33   Duhigg, Habit, p19

us into repeating a behaviour that creates a Reward. It's like a tiny 'program' in our brain that prompts us to carry out actions that should be good for us – such as finding fuel. A habit has three parts – a Trigger, an Action and a Reward.

Habit = Trigger → Action → Reward

The problem is that because our foods have evolved faster than we have, our Sugar Seeking Programme now prompts us to seek out refined sugar – even though this fuel is so concentrated that it overwhelms our ability to process it. Consuming sugar literally becomes a 'Bad Habit'. Our Sugar Seeking Programme is simply doing what it evolved to do – tracking the 'best' sources of sugar and encouraging us to consume them. Our brain can't tell the difference between a 'good' habit and a 'bad' one.[34]

Sugar Seeking Habits = Brain Spots An External Trigger → Tells Us To Find And Consume Sugar → We Feel Good

Habits are hard for us to control because when a trigger is activated, we don't decide whether to act on it or not.

---

34 Ibid, p20

The prompt that we get from our brain is not a question, 'Hey do you happen to fancy something sweet?', it's an instruction, 'Look for sugar and when you find some, eat it'. We automatically carry out the actions that are linked to a trigger – unless we use the conscious part of our brain to block the prompt from our unconscious. So we don't **choose** to consume sugar when our brain spots a trigger, but, if we can block the prompt from our unconscious, we can resist it. But, as you are well aware, this is not always easy to do.

The prompts from our unconscious can be hard to block because the conscious part of our brain uses more fuel than the unconscious part and sometimes, it just doesn't have enough fuel to be able to do this. So although we **can** resist our desire for sugar, we can't **always** resist our desire for sugar - which is why sugar is harder to resist when we are tired or stressed. And we are not usually keen to resist it because, if we don't act on the prompt from our brain, we feel that we are missing out. We feel good when we consume sugar but bad when we don't.

The stronger the trigger, the easier it is for the unconscious part of our brain to activate it – and the harder it is for the conscious part of our brain to block it. The habit pathway in our brain is like the pathway through a garden. If it is seldom used it becomes overgrown and difficult to walk down but if it is well used, a wide clear path emerges that is easy for our brain to follow. Consuming sugar is easy to do but hard to stop.

Sugar has a strong hold over us because we evolved in a world where sugar was in short supply so we evolved to consume sugar, not to resist it. The problem is that we are living in a world that is full of sugar with a brain that still believes that it is hard to find.

From the moment we first taste a sweet food, we create triggers that enable our brain to search for opportunities to consume more of it. Every time we act on these triggers, we add even more triggers to the Sugar Map in our head, giving our brain even more opportunities to prompt us to search for sugar. Those of us who create strong triggers can find that our desire for sugar grows and grows.

The amount of sugar that we consume can increase so much that a much more intense desire for it can appear. This is no longer just a fleeting 'Desire For Something Sweet' that pops into our head from time to time. It is a 'Need To Find Sugar Now!' We call this more intense feeling a 'craving'.

In the next chapter, we'll look at how sugar creates our cravings and we'll find out why they are even harder to resist.

3

Why We Get Cravings For Sugar

As we've seen, our desire for sugar is activated when our brain spots something that suggests that sugar may be close by. External Triggers tell our brain that we have an opportunity to find fuel.

External Triggers → Opportunity for Fuel → Desire

Our cravings are also created by triggers. But these triggers come from inside our body – so we'll call these 'Internal Triggers'. Our cravings are triggered, not by opportunity, but by need. When the unconscious part of our brain detects a drop in the blood sugar or neurotransmitters that it needs to function, it prompts us to find sugar because it sees sugar as a great source of fuel.

Internal Triggers → Need For Fuel → Craving

But ironically, it is sugar that creates the lack of fuel that our brain is trying to fix. In this chapter, we'll find out how sugar creates cravings by disrupting our blood sugar and neurotransmitters and we'll discover the reason why our cravings are so hard to resist.

How Sugar Disrupts Our Neurotransmitters

We've seen that our brain releases feel-good neurotransmitters to reward us for finding fuel and that sugar creates a surge of these neurotransmitters because it is such a concentrated fuel.

Although these surges in our neurotransmitters make us feel good initially, they are not normal and, if we create them too often, they can begin to make us feel bad because the extra neurotransmitters can overwhelm our brain. It's as though the messages that they create are being shouted in our brain instead of just being spoken at normal volume - so our brain takes action to stop this from happening.

It can't stop surges of neurotransmitters from being released when we consume sugar but it can stop the neurotransmitters from delivering their messages by switching off the receptors on our neurons. When the number of receptors is reduced, fewer neurotransmitters are able to find a receptor to hit so it becomes harder for the neurotransmitters to pass on their message. When there are fewer receptors available to listen to the message, it becomes less powerful - the volume is turned down. This process is called 'down regulation'.[35] Ironically when our brain reduces the number of receptors on our neurons to protect itself from the surges that are created by sugar, the amount of sugar that we consume actually goes up.

This happens because when the number of receptors in our brain is reduced, the reward that we get for finding fuel is also reduced. Sugar no longer makes us feel quite as good as it did before because there are fewer receptors to pick up the feel-good message. The fewer receptors we have, the more sugar we need to consume to release enough neurotransmitters to reach them all. So instead of eating a couple of cookies and putting the rest away, we now eat the entire packet.

The increase in the amount of sugar that we need to eat to feel good is known as our 'Tolerance' for sugar.[36] As our

---

35   Kharrazian, Datis. *Why Isn't My Brain Working?.* 1st ed.,p 75
36   Lustig, *Fat Chance,* p54

Tolerance increases sugar becomes more attractive and we eat more of it. This reduction in our receptors also means that foods that don't create a surge in our neurotransmitters become less appealing because the neurotransmitters that they release also hit fewer receptors. The reward that we get for consuming these foods becomes so small that we are no longer attracted to them - their feel-good message is turned down to a whisper. Foods that contain normal concentrations of sugar begin to seem boring and tasteless when compared foods that contain refined sugar so we begin to eat less of these foods.

Cake becomes more attractive than fruit because, once our brain has turned down the volume of the messages that are passed by our neurotransmitters, the messages that are created by sugar are at the right volume and the messages that are created by natural sugars aren't loud enough for our brain to hear. So now, if we don't consume sugar regularly, the receptors on our neurons receive too few neurotransmitters and the messages in our brain become too weak.

When the number of receptors is reduced, our brain prompts us to consume refined sugar so that we release enough neurotransmitters to keep the messages that they create at a normal level so we begin to get cravings for sugar that seem to appear from nowhere. Ironically, by trying to stop the messages from sugar from becoming overwhelming, our brain creates a need for sugar.

Normal Number Of Receptors	Reduced Number Of Receptors
Refined Sugars Create Too Many Neurotransmitters	Refined Sugars Create The Right Amount Of Neurotransmitters
Unrefined Sugars Create The Right Amount	Unrefined Sugars Don't Create Enough

We think that we crave sugar because it makes us feel good but, in reality, the opposite is true. We crave sugar because, if we don't consume it, our neurotransmitters fall and we feel bad. Cravings are not a sign that we love sugar. They are a sign that our brain is lacking the fuel that it needs to function.

This reduction in our receptors creates a vicious circle that keeps us hooked on sugar. We need to create surges in our neurotransmitters to hit enough of the remaining receptors to keep our brain happy. But when we do, our brain is forced to keep our receptors at a reduced level to stop these surges from creating messages that are too loud.

Surge In Our Neurotransmitters ↔ **Reduces The Number Of Receptors**

So sugar doesn't just create neurotransmitters, it creates an increased **need** for these neurotransmitters. Once we have added sugar to our diet, we need to keep consuming it because our brain becomes dependent on it.

Not only do we need to consume sugar regularly to keep our neurotransmitters at a normal level, we need to consume more sugar at times when our neurotransmitters need an extra boost. This means that when we are busy, sleep-deprived, stressed or upset our cravings for sugar increase. We call this 'comfort eating'.[37]

Our cravings for sugar can also increase in winter because the number of serotonin receptors in our brain naturally falls when there is less daylight. It is thought that this happens because, just as an increase in serotonin lifts our mood and increases our energy levels, a decrease does the opposite so we are able to conserve fuel at a time when the supply of food would normally have been limited.

However, this seasonal drop may have a more dramatic effect on our mood if the number of serotonin receptors in our brain has already been reduced by the sugar in our diet. Our cravings for sugar may increase because we are trying to boost our mood by increasing the amount of serotonin that is released in our brain. (And if you are a

---

37 'Sugar doesn't eliminate pain but it makes it more tolerable, although the more sugar the brain is exposed to the more it takes to control pain.' Gundry, *Diet Evolution,* p21

woman, your cravings may also increase before a period because this is the time when oestrogen, which stops the serotonin in your brain from being broken down, is at its lowest level).

So although sugar creates a temporary boost in our neurotransmitters, it has the opposite long term effect. When we consume sugar regularly, we need to release larger amounts of these neurotransmitters to keep our brain in balance. When we become dependent on sugar to keep our brain happy, our sugar consumption can increase so much that we can trigger a second survival programme.

We have actually inherited two programmes from our ancestors to help us to manage fuel. Our Sugar Seeking Programme, which helps us to find fuel, and our 'Sugar Rationing Programme', which controls what happens to it. If this second programme is triggered by the sugar in our diet, it can create drops in our blood sugar and neurotransmitters which can increase our cravings even more.

Let's look at what happens.

*

Our Sugar Rationing Programme

Our Sugar Rationing Programme determines whether the fuel that we consume is burned or stored. It enables us to store fuel by 'rationing' the amount of glucose that can enter our cells to be burned. Just like our Sugar Seeking Programme, this programme is controlled by the unconscious part of our brain so we are not aware of it. And, just like our Sugar Seeking Programme, it is controlled by triggers – some from inside our body (Internal Triggers), and some from the world around us (External Triggers).

The more active our Sugar Rationing Programme is the less glucose we burn and the more we store. It is activated when we hit puberty so that we burn less glucose and use more of it to build fat stores, such as hips and breasts. It is activated when we are pregnant so that we burn less glucose and use more of it to fuel the growth of a baby.[38] And it is also activated by changes in our food supply.

Our Sugar Rationing Programme can be triggered by both 'Feast' and 'Famine'. It is thought that extremes in our diet became triggers because this helped our ancestors to survive in a world that had a variable supply of fuel.

---

[38]   Castracane V. D. Et al., 'Serum Leptin in Nonpregnant and Pregnant Women and in Ols and New World Primates', Exp. Biol. Med. 230 (2005): 251-54 cited in Lustig, *Fat Chance*, p46

By reducing the amount of glucose that they burned in summer, when there was extra fuel available from fruit (the Feast Trigger), our ancestors were able to build fat stores to help them to survive the winter.[39] (The same programme is used by animals who store fat before going into hibernation). And by reducing the amount of glucose that they burned in the winter when there was little food (the Famine Trigger), our ancestors were able to survive by keeping the little fuel that was available for the organs that needed it most – like their brain.

Increased Fuel Supply – (Feast) Burn Less & Store Fuel For Winter

Reduced Fuel Supply – (Famine) Burn Less & Save Fuel For Vital Organs

Unlike our ancestors, we have plenty of food available throughout the year so we no longer need to build up fat stores in the summer or protect our organs from a lack of fuel in the winter. But, just like our Sugar Seeking Programme, our Sugar Rationing Programme is more active than ever because sugar mimics the extremes in our diet that switch this Programme on.

_____

39   Gundry, *Diet Evolution*, p32

How Sugar Creates The Feast Trigger

Sugar creates the Feast trigger because it is high in fructose. Our ancestors' diet was usually very low in fructose so a rise in the amount would have signalled the arrival of an increase in fuel in the form of fruit. This increase would have triggered our ancestors' Sugar Rationing Programme so that they could build fat stores for winter.

Although it is fructose that creates the trigger, it is glucose that the Programme affects because, as you may remember, fructose is used by very few cells so it is almost always turned into fat anyway. In fact, it is the visceral fat that is created by the fructose that actually gives the signal to switch this Programme on.

Fructose → Creates Visceral Fat → Switches On Sugar Rationing Programme → Burn Less Glucose → Store Fat For Winter

Once the supply of fruit ended, the amount of fructose in our ancestors' diet would have dropped so their stores of visceral fat would also have dropped. You may remember that visceral fat is kept around our organs for easy access so we burn this fat before we burn the fat that lies under our skin. When their visceral fat stores disappeared, their

Sugar Rationing Programme would have switched off and they would begin to burn glucose at a normal rate once again. Unlike our ancestors, we have a high level of fructose in our diet all year round so our Sugar Rationing Programme can be switched on permanently.

Many of us are continuously storing fat - preparing for a drop in our food supply that will never arrive. Forty percent of us who are a normal weight are carrying enough visceral fat to switch on our Sugar Rationing Programme. And this percentage can double for those of us who are overweight.[40]

In fact, the fructose that we get from sugar is more likely to trigger this Programme than the fructose that our ancestors got from fruit because sugar contains equal amounts of glucose and fructose and, as you may remember, glucose helps fructose to move out of our gut and into our bloodstream. This means that when the fructose comes from sugar more of it can be turned into visceral fat.

If you are female, the chances of triggering this Programme also increase with age because you will begin to store more visceral fat (and less subcutaneous fat) as your oestrogen level declines. Instead of storing fat on your hips and thighs you will begin to store it on your stomach. It is thought that the Feast trigger can also be activated by

40   Borysenko, Joan. *The Plantplus Diet Solution.* Chap 16

the uric acid that is produced when we process large amounts of fructose - and also by the bacteria in our gut that feed on fructose.

But sugar doesn't just create the Feast trigger. Perhaps more surprisingly it also creates the Famine trigger. The **high level of fructose** in sugar tells our brain that there is extra fuel available and that we should reduce the amount of fuel that we burn so that we can create fat stores for winter. But the **fast-digesting glucose** in sugar tells our brain to reduce the amount of fuel that we burn because it tricks our brain into thinking that our fuel stores are on the verge of running out. The message that sugar gives our brain is this – 'The bad news is that you are running out of fuel but the good news is that there is plenty of fuel available so reduce what you burn and keep eating'. Let's find out how sugar creates the Famine Trigger.

How Sugar Creates The Famine Trigger

The trigger for Famine is created by a hormone called 'leptin'. Leptin is created by our fat cells and it circulates in our bloodstream. The more fat we have, the more leptin we make. When food was scarce our ancestors would have burned their fat stores for fuel so the amount of leptin in their bloodstream would have decreased. This drop in leptin would have triggered their Sugar Rationing Programme – reducing the amount of glucose that their cells could burn so that the little fuel that was available could be used by the organs that needed it most.[41]

Low Fat Stores → Low Leptin → Burn Less Glucose → Save Fuel For Vital Organs

Using only a minimal amount of fuel and storing any excess as fat enabled our ancestors to maintain their fat stores for as long as possible and to rebuild them when the supply of food improved. As their fat stores increased, the amount of leptin in their bloodstream would have risen. This would have turned their Sugar Rationing Programme off so that they would begin to burn glucose at a normal rate once again.

Happily, most of us are far from starvation.[42] We have plenty of stored fat and a more than adequate supply of leptin. But the sugar in our diet can mimic the Famine trigger because although we have plenty of leptin in our bloodstream, our brain can't see it.

41   Energy expenditure can reduce by 20%. Leibel, Rudolph L. et al "Changes In Energy Expenditure Resulting From Altered Body Weight". New England Journal of Medicine 332.10 (1995): 621-628. Web. Cited in Lustig, *Fat Chance* p40
42   World Health Organisation, Fact Sheet: Obesity and Overweight (2011), cited in Lustig, *Fat Chance*, p5

We've seen that when we create a surge of glucose in our bloodstream, we release a surge of insulin to move the glucose safely into our cells. The problem is that insulin can block the leptin signal to our brain. So when we have a large amount of insulin in our bloodstream, our brain thinks that our fat stores are dangerously low, regardless of how much fat we actually have. This is known as 'Leptin Resistance'.

Surge Of Glucose → Surge Of Insulin → Leptin Signal Is Blocked → Sugar Rationing Programme Switched On → Burn Less Glucose

There are times when we want insulin to block the leptin signal. It is an increase in insulin that activates our Sugar Rationing Programme when we hit puberty or become pregnant. You may remember that it is insulin that tells our cells to divide and grow – and this includes our fat cells. Once we have made the transition to adulthood or given birth, our insulin level drops and our Sugar Rationing Programme switches off. But, if our insulin level is high because of the sugar in our diet, our Sugar Rationing Programme can stay active because our fat stores are always hidden from our brain.

By changing from sugars that are 'Low and Slow' (low

in fructose and containing slow-digesting glucose) to sugars that are the 'High and Fast', we have created a diet that keeps our Sugar Rationing Programme permanently switched on. Our diet is always 'extreme' because when our Sugar Programmes evolved, refined carbohydrates, such as sugar, were not part of our diet.

And it's not just the sugar in our own diet that can switch this Programme on. The sugar in our mother's diet can do this too. When the Programme is activated in a mother-to-be, it is also activated in her baby so that both mother and baby can create fat stores to help them to survive the winter if there is extra fuel available and the vital organs in both can be protected if there is little fuel available. This means that, if our mother had a high sugar diet, our Sugar Rationing Programme may have been switched on before we were even born.[43]When our Sugar Rationing Programme is active our cravings for sugar can become more intense. To find out why we need to look at how our Sugar Rationing Programme works.

How Our Sugar Rationing Programme Works

Our Sugar Rationing Programme reduces the amount of glucose that our cells can burn by switching off the

---

43   Lustig, *Fat Chance*, p80

insulin receptors that unlock our cells to let glucose inside. When our insulin receptors are switched on and glucose can get into our cells easily, we say that our cells are 'sensitive' to insulin. When these receptors switch off and our cells begin to refuse to let glucose in, we say that they are 'resistant' to insulin. The more resistant our cells become the less glucose we burn. The receptors on our cells work like valves, not on/off switches, so the amount of glucose that can be moved into the cell works on a sliding scale.

Insulin Sensitive → → → → Insulin Resistant

Burn More → → → → → → → Burn Less

When the insulin receptors on our cells switch off, not all of our cells shut glucose out to the same degree because some of our cells need insulin to move glucose into the cell, but others don't need it at all. Our liver and muscle cells are most dependent on insulin so these cells have a drastic cut in their fuel supply. But cells that need a constant supply of glucose, like our brain, can simply absorb the glucose that they need directly from our bloodstream so the fuel supply to these cells is never reduced.

Our fat cells are somewhere in the middle.[44] They need insulin to move glucose into the cell but they are happier to let it in than our muscle and liver cells.

Least Dependent $\rightarrow$ $\rightarrow$ $\rightarrow$ $\rightarrow$ **Most Dependent**
On Insulin   **On Insulin**

Brain, Nerve & $\rightarrow$ **Fat Cells** $\rightarrow$ **Liver &**
Red Blood Cells   **Muscle Cells**

This means that when the insulin receptors on our cells begin to switch off, less glucose is able to enter our muscle and liver cells to be burned. This leaves the glucose circulating in our bloodstream to be absorbed by the cells that need it the most - like our brain cells. If there is any glucose left over, after these cells have taken what they need, our fat cells are happy to let it in. Reducing the amount of fuel that we burn in this way allows us to prioritise the fuel supply to our vital organs when there is little fuel available and to build our fat stores when there is a lot of fuel available.

However, this fuel rationing system evolved before refined sugar appeared in our diet. If we consume sugar

---

44   Gedgaudas, *Primal Body*, p141

whilst our Sugar Rationing Programme is active the surges that are created in our blood sugar and neurotransmitters become much higher because it is much harder to move the excess glucose out of our bloodstream and into our cells when our liver and muscle cells are no longer as willing to burn it off.

Foods that create a moderate rise in our blood sugar when our cells are happy to let glucose inside begin to create surges in our blood sugar when they are not. And foods that create surges in our blood sugar begin to create even bigger surges in our blood sugar.

So sugar doesn't just create surges in our blood sugar that our ancestors didn't experience, it also reduces our ability to control these surges because although we are bombarding our cells with fuel, we are telling our cells to reduce the amount of glucose that they burn.

When the surges in our blood sugar become more dramatic, our cravings for sugar can become more intense because these surges can also begin to produce drops.

Let's find out why this happens.

How Blood Sugar Surges Become Blood Sugar Drops

Having a high level of glucose in our bloodstream is not good news because, as we saw in Chapter 1, glucose can damage our cells by binding with proteins (glycation). The higher our blood sugar becomes, the more opportunity the glucose has to cause harm. And ironically, the cells that our Sugar Rationing Programme evolved to protect are the ones that are most at risk because these are the cells that absorb glucose directly from our bloodstream.

Our ancestors didn't experience surges in their blood sugar so we have not evolved a way to shut off the fuel supply to these cells. This means that they are flooded with glucose whenever our blood sugar level surges. Glycation is the primary cause of brain degeneration as we age - possibly leading to dementia and Alzheimers (which is created by tangles of glycated proteins that stick together).[45]

To protect these cells from harm we have to move the excess glucose out of our bloodstream and into our cells - even if the receptors on our cells don't want to let it in - so our pancreas releases more insulin to force these cells to respond.

The amount of insulin that we need to release to move the glucose safely into our cells depends on the amount of glucose we have consumed, the speed that it is reaching our bloodstream and the reluctance of our cells to allow the glucose inside. The higher the surge in our blood sugar and the greater the resistance of our cells, the more insulin we need to release.

---

45   Kharrazian, *Brain*, p70-71

Insulin Needed = Amount of Glucose + Speed That It Arrives + Cells' Reluctance To Let It In

However, we haven't evolved the ability to be able to precisely calculate the amount of insulin that we release in this way because the amount of glucose in our ancestors' diet was never very high and it varied very little. The amount of insulin that we actually release is based on the amount that has worked on previous occasions. We simply release a surge of insulin in response to a surge of glucose and, if this fails to clear the glucose, then we release a second smaller burst of it to finish the job.

Not only does the amount of glucose in our bloodstream vary enormously depending on what we have eaten, but our cells' resistance to insulin also varies dramatically because it is affected by other hormones in our body. For example, cortisol, the hormone that gives us our 'get up and go' in the mornings, increases our cells' resistance to insulin so we need to release more insulin to move glucose into our cells in the morning than we do later in the day.

This means that it is easy for too much insulin to be released and for too much glucose to be cleared from our bloodstream. When this happens, the surge in our blood sugar can become a drop that can trigger a sugar craving. Remember it's not insulin's 'job' to control surges in our blood sugar because we are not supposed to have surges in our blood sugar.[46]

How Drops In Our Blood Sugar Can Trigger Cravings

Drops in our blood sugar can trigger our cravings because our brain is very sensitive to the amount of glucose in our bloodstream. As we've seen, our brain absorbs the glucose that it needs directly from our blood so if there is even a slight fall in the amount of glucose that is available, our brain will take action to boost it. We usually raise our blood sugar by releasing a hormone called 'glucagon' from our pancreas to turn some of the glucose that we have stored as glycogen back into glucose.

However, glucagon can't do its job if the drop in our blood sugar is the result of too much insulin being released because glucagon is blocked by insulin.[47] Remember, insulin is released when we need to gain weight so as well as blocking the leptin signal to our brain so that we store more of the glucose that we consume, it locks the glucose that we have already stored (not just as glucagon but also as fat) into our cells. When glucagon is blocked, we can boost

---

46   We have evolved to increase blood sugar not lower it. See Gedgaudas, *Primal Body*, p128
47   Ibid, p139

our blood sugar by releasing stress hormones but this can make us feel anxious and irritable.

It is thought that these drops in our blood sugar can create cravings for two reasons. Firstly, our brain is prompting us to look for sugar to boost our blood sugar level so that it has access to the fuel that it needs.

Secondly, our brain is prompting us to look for sugar to boost our feel-good neurotransmitters to counteract the effect of the stress hormones that we have released.

Low Blood Sugar / → Need For Fuel → Craving Neurotransmitters

Cravings can begin to appear after we have eaten sugar (or another refined carbohydrate) because the surge in our blood sugar that results can lead to too much insulin being released - turning the surge into a drop. Cravings can also begin to appear between meals because, when our insulin levels are high, we can't unlock the fuel that we have stored to maintain our blood sugar until the next meal. We may also begin to feel irritable, anxious and light-headed if we don't eat regularly.[48] And of course, when we consume sugar in response to a craving, we can

---

48   If we don't eat we should experience hunger not irritability, dizziness, brain fog, fatigue, brain fog, jitteriness or mood swings. Ibid, p131

create another surge in our blood sugar which can lead to another drop – and another craving.

Our cravings for sugar are not normal. They appear because, although sugar is a concentrated fuel, it's not a fuel that suits us. Our Sugar Rationing Programme hasn't evolved to be able to cope with refined carbohydrates. Ironically it is our brain's attempt to protect us from the glucose surges that sugar creates, by reducing the number of receptors on our neurons and by releasing surges of insulin to move excess glucose out of our bloodstream, that creates the cravings that drive the amount of sugar in our diet up and up.

Sugar doesn't just create surges in our blood sugar, it also reduces our body's ability to return our blood sugar to a normal level. And, over time, the surges can grow worse because sugar doesn't just turn our Sugar Rationing Programme on, it also turns it up - resulting in an increase in our cravings.

How Our Cravings Increase

Sugar activates our Sugar Rationing Programme because, as we've seen, it creates both the Feast trigger (visceral fat created by fructose) and the Famine trigger (high levels of insulin created in response to fast-digesting glucose).

The more sugar we consume, the more visceral fat and insulin we create so the stronger these triggers become. Remember our Sugar Rationing Programme isn't an on/off programme, it works on a scale so as the triggers become stronger our cells become more and more reluctant to let glucose inside.

The harder it is to move the excess glucose out of our bloodstream and into our cells, the higher the surges in our blood sugar become and the more insulin we need to release to force our cells to respond. This creates a vicious circle that turns our Sugar Rationing Programme up and up because the more insulin we release, the stronger the Famine trigger becomes which means that more glucose is moved into our fat cells. And the more fat we create, the stronger the Feast trigger becomes - because when we move the glucose into our fat cells, we also move it into our visceral fat cells.

We Consume Sugar → We Release Insulin → The Insulin Blocks Our Leptin Signal (Increasing The Famine Trigger) → We Store More Of The Glucose As (Visceral) Fat (Increasing The Feast Trigger) → Our Cells Become More Resistant To Insulin → We Release More Insulin To Make Our Cells Respond

The more active our Sugar Rationing Programme, the less responsive our cells become and the more insulin we release in response to glucose. This creates ups and downs in our blood sugar that are increasingly dramatic and can result in more frequent (and more intense) cravings. Firstly, because our brain has to prompt us to find sugar more frequently to prop up our falling blood sugar. Secondly, because as the ups and downs in our blood sugar become more dramatic, the ups and downs in our neurotransmitters follow suit so we need to consume more sugar just to keep our neurotransmitters at a normal level.

We've seen that a surge in our blood sugar creates a surge in our neurotransmitters that switches off the receptors on our neurons - creating an increased need for these neurotransmitters. So when the surges in our blood sugar and neurotransmitters become more dramatic, our brain shuts down even more of the receptors on our neurons.

We Consume Sugar → We Create Feast & Famine Triggers → Insulin Receptors On Our Cells Switch Off → There Is More Disruption To Our Blood Sugar & Neurotransmitters → Receptors On Our Neurons Switch Off → Our Cravings Increase → We Consume More Sugar

The fewer receptors there are for our neurotransmitters to hit, the more sugar we need to consume to ensure that we hit enough of the remaining receptors to keep our brain in balance. The more sugar we consume, the worse our cravings become.

As our Sugar Rationing Programme becomes more and more active, we move further up the scale of insulin resistance. Eventually, our cells can become so resistant to insulin that they may refuse to let glucose into the cell even when our pancreas is releasing as much insulin as it can. When this happens we may only be able to move glucose into our cells if we take additional insulin. We call this 'Type 2 Diabetes'. (Type 1 occurs if the cells in our pancreas are no longer able to create insulin). Studies suggest that for every 100 calories of sugar in our daily diet, our risk of developing diabetes rises by 0.9%.[49]

Sensitive To Insulin → Insulin Resistant → Pre-Diabetes → Diabetes

We don't all reach the top of the scale and develop diabetes but we tend to move up the scale more quickly as we age because we lose muscle cells (so we have fewer

---

49   Lustig, *Fat Chance*, p126

cells that can burn off excess glucose) and we create more visceral fat (so the signal to store glucose becomes stronger). But each generation seems to be progressing up the scale faster than the last.[50]

More of us may be developing diabetes because, if our Sugar Rationing Programme was activated before birth, the amount of insulin that we need to release to force our cells to respond to glucose is set at a higher level. But the number of insulin-producing cells that develop in our pancreas is set at a lower level (because a high level of glucose in our bloodstream before birth stops these cells from developing). This means that we need to produce **more** insulin to force our cells to respond but we actually produce **less** of it - so our cells stop responding to insulin (and we can develop diabetes) faster than someone who has a lot of these cells.[51]

Now that we have had a high sugar diet for several generations, each generation may be more susceptible to sugar cravings than the last because it is more likely that our mother had a high sugar diet and that our cells became resistant to insulin before we were born. The majority of people today release double the amount of insulin in response to glucose than people did 30 years

50   'Teens with diabetes used to be unheard of; now they are one-third of all new diagnoses of diabetes.' Ibid, p4
51   Ibid p80

ago, regardless of their weight.[52] Our ancestors changed sugar, but sugar may now be changing us.

*

Refined carbohydrates helped our ancestors to survive the winter because they provided them with extra fuel. But the High and Fast sugars in our diet can do the opposite. Instead of providing us with extra fuel they can create a constant **need** for fuel. Sugar creates a surge in our neurotransmitters that makes us feel good, but, as we've seen, this surge increases our need for neurotransmitters creating a constant need for sugar.

And if we consume enough sugar to activate our Sugar Rationing Programme (and we are storing fuel instead of burning it), our brain has to continually prompt us to find sugar to prop up our blood sugar because, despite all the fuel that we are consuming, we keep running out.

The problem is that once this programme has been activated it is hard to switch it off because sugar keeps it active and, as I'm sure you are aware, our cravings for sugar are hard to resist.

Let's find out why.

---

52   Ibid, p47

Why Our Cravings Are Hard To Resist

The unconscious part of our brain prompts us to look for sugar when it spots a drop in our blood sugar or neurotransmitters (an Internal Trigger), in the same way that it prompts us to look for sugar when it spots something in the world around us that signals that sugar may be close by (an External Trigger).

In both cases, we automatically begin to search for sugar unless we can use the conscious part of our brain to block this prompt. But the Internal Triggers that create our cravings are usually much harder to resist than the External Triggers that create our desire for sugar because the conscious part of our brain needs fuel to be able to block the prompts from our unconscious and our cravings are triggered when we need fuel. It is much harder to resist a need for fuel than it is to resist a desire for it. Remember, the conscious part of your brain needs **more** fuel to function than the unconscious part. If we lack the fuel that we need to block the prompt from our unconscious we find ourselves consuming sugar in response to a craving – even if we would prefer not to.

Internal Triggers (Cravings) Caused By Lack Of Fuel = Hard To Resist / Dependent On Fuel Supply

External Triggers aren't created by drops in our fuel supply so the conscious part of our brain usually has the fuel that it needs to block these triggers.

External Triggers Caused By Environment/Activities = Easier To Resist / Independent Of Fuel Supply

But they can become just as hard to block if they coincide with a lack of fuel. For example, if we are shopping our brain may spot one or more of the triggers that it has created for sugar. We will be able to block the prompts that these triggers create if the conscious part of our brain has the fuel that it needs to do this but we will act on them if it doesn't - which is why it is always harder to resist buying sugary treats if we shop on an empty stomach.

Our External Triggers also become harder to block when our Sugar Rationing Programme is active because, when we begin to suffer drops in our blood sugar and neurotransmitters, the conscious part of our brain lacks the fuel that it needs to block these triggers for more of the time. The more active this programme is, the harder it becomes to resist the prompts that our brain creates in response to our environment and our activities - which increases the amount of sugar in our diet even further.

Our sugar consumption can begin to spiral out of control because, when our Sugar Rationing Programme turns on, our Sugar Seeking Programme turns up. We can begin to track sugar like a heat-seeking missile. In the next chapter, we'll find out how our Sugar Seeking Programme and our Sugar Rationing Programme have evolved to work together to increase the amount of sugar in our diet and we'll find out why sugar sends these programmes into overdrive.

4

Why We Lose Control Of Our Sugar Consumption

We've seen that we have two Programmes to help us to find and use fuel. Our Sugar Seeking Programme which enables us to track and predict sources of sugar and our Sugar Rationing Programme which determines how much of the sugar we burn and how much we store. These Programmes evolved to work together. When our Sugar Seeking Programme is able to find large amounts of sugar (the Feast trigger), our Sugar Rationing Programme swings into action so that we can store it.

Our Sugar Seeking Programme → Activates Our Sugar Rationing Programme

And when our Sugar Rationing Programme is active and we need more fuel, to get us through pregnancy or puberty or to survive a Famine, our Sugar Seeking Programme shifts up a gear so that we can find and consume more of it - so an increase in one programme creates an increase in the other.

Our Sugar Rationing Programme → Activates Our Sugar Seeking Programme

The problem is that when these programmes are triggered by the refined sugar in our diet, they can increase rapidly sending our sugar consumption spiralling out of control. In this chapter, we're going to look at how these programmes have evolved to work together and we'll find out why refined sugar sends these programmes into overdrive.

We've already seen how our Sugar Rationing Programme can be activated by large amounts of sugar in our diet so now let's see how our Sugar Rationing Programme turns up our Sugar Seeking Programme by making sugar more attractive.

Why Sugar Becomes More Attractive

We've seen that the insulin receptors on our cells switch off when our Sugar Rationing Programme is active so that we can store more of the glucose that we consume.

But this Programme doesn't just reduce the amount of glucose that we burn, it also increases the amount that we eat. We consume larger portions of sugar when our Sugar Rationing Programme is switched on because the reward that we get when we consume sugar lasts for a longer period of time. Our Sugar Rationing Programme activates our Sugar Seeking Programme because it doesn't just tell us to 'Burn Less', it also tells us to 'Eat More'.

Sugar Rationing Programme = Burn Less + Eat More

As you may remember, it is dopamine, the neuro-transmitter that activates our Reward Centre, that creates the feelings of pleasure that we get when we consume sugar. The length of time that this feeling of pleasure lasts is determined by leptin, the hormone that is made by our fat cells. When glucose reaches our bloodstream and we release insulin to move it into our cells, we also release leptin.

The leptin tells our brain to stop releasing dopamine so we stop getting pleasure from the food that we are eating. When we are rewarded for eating, we eat and when the reward stops, we stop. So leptin doesn't just tell our brain how much fat we have in storage, it also helps to regulate our appetite.

The longer the reward lasts, the more we eat.

We Consume Sugar → Dopamine Is Released (Reward) → Glucose Reaches Our Bloodstream → Insulin & Leptin Are Released → Dopamine Release Stops (No Reward) → We Stop Eating

When our Sugar Rationing Programme is active the reward that we get when we consume sugar lasts longer because the leptin signal that switches it off becomes weaker.

As we saw in Chapter 3, the leptin signal can become weaker either because we have used up our fat stores and there is less leptin in our body which happens when we are starving (Low Leptin) or it can become weaker because the signal is blocked by a high level of insulin which happens if we are pregnant, going through puberty or there is a lot of sugar in our diet (Leptin Resistance).

Let's look at each of these in turn.

Low Leptin

If we have low levels of leptin because we have used up our fat stores, the signal that switches off the reward for finding fuel becomes weaker because there is less leptin for our body to release. The reward lasts longer so we eat more. Our appetite increases dramatically - we become ravenous - because we need to increase our fuel intake to survive.

Low Fat Stores → Low Leptin → Dopamine Released For Longer → Increased Reward → We Eat More

In fact, the amount of leptin that circulates in our bloodstream doesn't just drop when we have lost our fat stores, it drops as soon as the amount that we eat drops. We evolved in a world where fuel was hard to find so it would have been foolish to wait until our fat stores had gone before increasing our appetite. By making the leptin signal responsive to changes in our diet, as well as changes in our fat stores, our brain is able to take action to increase our fuel supply straight away.

As soon as our fuel supply goes down, the reward that we get for finding fuel goes up so that we are motivated to consume more of it. This is why we find it so hard to stick to a low-calorie diet.

Leptin Resistance

When the leptin signal to our brain is blocked by a high level of insulin, the reward that we get when we eat lasts longer because our brain can't see the signal that switches it off[53].

High Insulin → Blocks Leptin → Dopamine Released For Longer → Increased Reward → We Eat More

This is what happens if we are pregnant, going through puberty or if we have a high sugar diet. Pregnant women eat 'for two' and teenagers eat like a plague of locusts because they need extra fuel to grow. If we have a high sugar diet, we don't need any extra fuel but our brain thinks that we do because the insulin that is released in response to the fast-digesting glucose stops our brain from seeing our fat stores. Our appetite increases and we store more of the sugar that we eat because our brain is trying to 'rebuild' our fat stores.

Leptin resistance should only create a temporary increase in our appetite because our Sugar Rationing Programme shouldn't be continuously active. If this programme has been triggered by famine, pregnancy or puberty, it switches off and our appetite returns to normal

---

53   Lustig, *Fat Chance*, p52

once we have rebuilt our fat stores, given birth or reached adulthood. The problem is that when our Sugar Rationing Programme is triggered by high levels of refined sugar in our diet it never switches off so our appetite stays permanently high.

When our appetite increases we don't just eat more food, we eat more sugary food because the reward that we get from refined sugar is the longest lasting of all. As you may remember, foods that contain fructose are more rewarding because we release the leptin that tells our brain to shut off the reward when we release insulin. And we release insulin in response to glucose but not in response to fructose so the more fructose a food contains the longer the reward lasts and the more we can eat.[54] You may remember that animals binge on fruit (which has the highest natural concentration of fructose and that sugar contains a lot more fructose than even the sweetest fruit).

When our Sugar Rationing Programme is active the reward that we get from sugar lasts even longer than usual because the signal to switch off the reward is not only being delayed by fructose, it is also being blocked by insulin. High sugar foods become even more attractive because the reward that we get from these foods increases but foods that contain (normal) lower concentrations of

54   Gundry, *Diet Evolution*, p32

sugar become less attractive because the reward that we get from these foods decreases.

We've already seen that consuming sugar reduces our attraction to these foods because sugar creates surges in our neurotransmitters that switch off the receptors on our neurons making it harder for the smaller amounts of neurotransmitter that are released by low sugar foods to be able to find a receptor to pass on their feel-good message. But low sugar foods become even less rewarding when dopamine is released in our brain for longer because our brain responds by switching off even more of our dopamine receptors - so the chance of finding a receptor to hit reduces even further.

By making sugar even more rewarding when our Sugar Rationing Programme is active, our brain is able to direct us to the most concentrated sources of fuel and to increase the amount that we eat. It makes sense for our brain to do this because it thinks that we have an increased need for fuel. However, if this programme has been activated by refined sugar, a vicious circle is created because our Sugar Rationing Programme motivates us to consume more sugar and sugar keeps our Sugar Rationing Programme switched on - so our appetite for sugar stays permanently high even though we don't need the extra fuel.

The amount of sugar in our diet begins to climb, not only because we are consuming larger portions of it, but also because the increased reward means that we are more motivated to seek it out. In other words, our Sugar Rationing Programme turns up our Sugar Seeking Programme. Let's find out why this happens.

Why Our Sugar Consumption Begins To Climb

In Chapter 2 we saw how the dopamine that we release in response to sugar activates our memory so that we create External Triggers that enable our brain to find sugar again in the future. Our brain tracks foods that are high in sugar because these foods create large rewards and strong triggers. So, when we begin to release more dopamine in response to sugar, we don't just get a larger reward from it, we also create stronger triggers for it. And the stronger the trigger, the more easily our brain is able to activate it.

Our Sugar Seeking Programme is always on the lookout for the most concentrated sources of sugar - and we always create stronger triggers for these foods - but the process becomes more intense when our Sugar Rationing Programme is active because we get more of a reward for sugar.

The amount of sugar in our diet begins to climb because each time we come into contact with a new food that is a concentrated source of sugar – a new flavour of cereal that we sample at our local supermarket, a new type of cookie that we are given by a friend or a new dessert on the menu at our favourite restaurant - we update the Sugar Map in our head to show these new sources of fuel.

Our ancestors didn't have access to refined sugars so they would only ever have replaced the low sugar foods on their Sugar Map with other low sugar foods but over time, the low sugar foods on our Sugar Map can be replaced by high sugar ones. And once a high sugar food has been added to the Map, it usually stays on the Map because it is usually a (processed) food that is available to us all year round.

This means that the Map in our head gets bigger and bigger - giving our brain more and more opportunities to prompt us to consume sugar. In contrast, the Sugar Map in our ancestors' brain would have changed slowly in time with the seasons and it would have remained small because as some foods came into season, others would have disappeared.

It's not just refined sugar that we find more attractive, foods that are high in fast-digesting glucose become more attractive too so the amount of starchy carbohydrates in our diet can also begin to increase.

For example, if you work late one night a week and are too tired to go home and cook, you might just grab some hot chicken and a prepared salad on your way home. But, if the plain chicken has sold out one day, you may buy the chicken in the crunchy breadcrumb coating instead. The breadcrumb coating makes the chicken a more concentrated source of fuel (because flour is a source of fast-digesting glucose) so you will release more feel-good neurotransmitters in your brain in response to the crunchy chicken. When you stop to buy chicken the following week, your brain will spot the triggers that it created for the crunchy chicken on your last visit and it will prompt you to buy it.

It's unlikely that you will want to resist the prompt from your unconscious because the crunchy chicken creates more of a reward in your brain than the plain chicken. But, even if you do want to block the prompt, you will only be able to do so if the conscious part of your brain has enough fuel to be able to do this – which it may not after you have finished a long day at work. When you buy the crunchy chicken a second time, you strengthen the triggers in your brain so they become even harder to block on your next visit. After a few weeks, you have 'got into the habit' of buying the crunchy chicken and you buy it without a second thought.

Now let's say that the following month when you stop to buy your usual crunchy chicken and salad, the shop is offering free spicy fries with all purchases of chicken.

Potatoes contain a lot more glucose than your usual salad so the fries will create a bigger reward in your brain. On your next visit, your brain will spot the triggers that it created for the fries and it will prompt you to buy them instead of the salad.

You will only buy the salad if you are able to use the conscious part of your brain to block the prompt from your unconscious. But, once again, you may not want to block this prompt because you get more pleasure from the fries than you do from the salad. Every time you buy the fries, you strengthen the triggers even more so the prompt from your brain becomes even harder to block. Over time, your habit of buying plain chicken and salad once a week becomes a habit of buying crunchy chicken and fries.

When the triggers on our Sugar Map change, our diet changes because the foods that we choose to eat are the ones that appear on this Map. When our brain spots one of the triggers that it has created, it prompts us to look for the food that is linked to that trigger and we automatically begin to seek it out - unless we can use the conscious part of our brain to block the prompt.

As we've seen it's not usually hard to block these External Triggers because they are activated by things in our environment and not by a need for fuel so the conscious part of our brain normally has the fuel that it needs to block them. The problem is that we don't usually want to block them because these high sugar foods create more pleasure. The more often we act on the prompt that is created by a trigger, the stronger the trigger becomes and the stronger the trigger becomes the more often we act on it - which is why we tend to eat the same foods over and over again. Our diet is simply a collection of all the habits that we have created that help us to find fuel which is why we talk about our 'dietary (or eating) habits'.

Dietary Habits = (External) Trigger → Action (Eat) → Reward (Fuel)

Each of us has a unique diet because each of us has created a unique network of External Triggers – depending on the foods that we have come into contact with in the past. One hundred vegetarians will have one hundred different vegetarian diets for example.

When the reward that we get for consuming sugar increases our diet begins to change because our brain begins to drive us more insistently towards the foods that are highest in sugar. Of course, we don't realise that we are creating stronger triggers for the foods that contain the most sugar. We just think that we 'prefer' the taste of them. One of the reasons that the 'hidden' sugars in packaged foods are such a problem is that, when our Sugar Rationing

Programme is active, these are the foods that we are unconsciously drawn towards.

But you may find that if you were to take a selection box containing mini packets of breakfast cereal or a box of chocolates and you were to rate them from your most to least favourite, those with the most sugar would be at the top (those caramel filled chocolates and the frosted flakes) and those with the least would be at the bottom (those dark chocolates with nuts and the boring grown-up cereals).

Our sugar consumption can increase so much that we can end up on the 'Sugar In Everything' diet where virtually all the foods that we eat - from our morning cereal to our lunch time baked potato, to our evening pasta – create surges in our blood sugar. (I call this the 'Sugar In Everything' diet because many of us are convinced that sugar is impossible to escape because it seems to be 'In Everything'. It's not in everything but it may be in everything that your brain prompts you to eat).

When our Sugar Rationing Programme is active, our Sugar Seeking Programme creates stronger triggers for sugar and our diet begins to change because this is what is supposed to happen. Our Sugar Rationing Programme increases the reward that we get from sugar because, when this programme is active, our brain thinks that we need to find more fuel. We evolved in a world where fuel was hard to find so our sugar programmes have evolved to work together to **maximise** our fuel consumption. The problem is that we have something that our ancestors didn't have that sends this process into overdrive – cravings.

Once we begin to search for sugar in response to our cravings, our Sugar Map explodes and our sugar consumption shoots up.

Let's look at how this happens.

How Our Cravings Drive Up Our Sugar Consumption

Our cravings drive up our sugar consumption because, instead of just creating triggers for high sugar foods that cross our path by chance, they drive us to actively search for new sources of sugar – often several times a day.

For example, if you happen to be in a shopping mall when you get a craving for sugar, you will use the External Triggers that you have already created to help you to find sugar. Your brain is good at finding new sources of sugar because it has already created many triggers that will tell it where to look. The scent of baking may draw you to a doughnut stand that you hadn't noticed before. If you buy a doughnut to satisfy your craving, you will create strong External Triggers for the doughnut and it will be added to the Sugar Map in your brain.

The next time you visit the mall, the External Triggers that you created on your last visit will be activated, so even though you may not have a craving for sugar this time, the idea that you 'just fancy a doughnut' pops into your head. If you 'treat' yourself to another doughnut, you will strengthen these triggers (and create new ones) so the desire to buy a doughnut will be stronger on your next visit. Treating yourself to a doughnut when you visit the mall soon becomes a habit. By consuming a doughnut in response to a need for sugar, you have created a desire for sugar that will appear every time you visit the mall.

We Eat A Doughnut $\rightarrow$ **The Desire For A Doughnut**
At The Mall In Response   **Appears On Every Trip**
To A Craving   **To The Mall**

Our cravings, or Internal Triggers, increase our sugar consumption because they are the driving force behind the creation of huge numbers of External Triggers for high sugar foods[55] that lead us back to sugar again and again - long after the craving that originally created them has gone. When we consume sugar in response to a craving, we change our eating habits.

The more of these triggers we add to our Sugar Map,

---

55   Duhigg, *Habits*, p33

the more opportunities our brain has to find sugar - so our desire for 'something sweet' begins to appear more and more frequently.

Internal Triggers → External Triggers For Sugar (Cravings) (Eating Habits)

But it doesn't stop there because, when we have a craving, our brain searches for foods that create surges in our blood sugar so we are actively creating External Triggers for foods that can disrupt our blood sugar and create more cravings in the future. For example, if you get into the habit of treating yourself to a doughnut when you arrive at the mall, you can create a surge and crash in your blood sugar that can trigger a craving a couple of hours into your visit.

Trip To The Mall → Consume A Doughnut (Desire) → Blood Sugar Surge & Crash → Craving

We think that our cravings appear randomly and that they come from nowhere but they don't. The drops in our blood sugar and neurotransmitters that trigger our cravings are created by our dietary habits. Any food that creates a surge in our blood sugar can create a craving, not just the sweet ones. So if we swap from a weekly meal of plain chicken and salad to one of crunchy chicken and fries, we may create a surge and crash in our blood sugar that prompts us to grab a sweet treat for dessert. So our habit of eating chicken and salad once a week eventually becomes a habit of eating crunchy chicken, fries and cheesecake.

*

Our sugar consumption spirals out of control because our cravings change our diet (by creating triggers for high sugar foods) into a diet that creates cravings (because these foods create surges and crashes in our blood sugar).

Cravings → **Triggers For** → **Cravings**
For Sugar **High Sugar Foods** **For Sugar**

Or to put it another way, our Internal Triggers create External Triggers and our External Triggers create Internal Triggers so the more sugar we consume, the more we crave.

Internal → **External** → **Internal**
Triggers **Triggers** **Triggers**

This cycle repeats itself over and over again. If you buy some chocolate to eat on the way home from the mall in response to the craving that you created when you ate the doughnut, you will create External Triggers for the chocolate too.

So when you visit the mall in the future, your brain will prompt you to buy a doughnut to eat when you arrive and a chocolate bar to eat on the way home. And the chocolate that you eat on the way home may create another surge and crash in your blood sugar that prompts another craving later on.

Our External Triggers are supposed to exist and we are supposed to eat more high fuel foods when our Sugar Rationing Programme is active. However, the cravings or Internal Triggers that push this process into overdrive are not supposed to exist. They are created because sugar creates surges in our blood sugar and neurotransmitters that are not supposed to be there.

Our sugar consumption can also climb because our cravings have a second effect on our diet. They don't just change what we eat, they also change when we eat. Let's find out how our cravings change our eating patterns.

*

How Cravings Change Our Eating Patterns

We've seen that when we consume sugar we create External Triggers that link the sugar to the place that we found it, the activity that we were carrying out and even to the time of day so that our brain can prompt us to search for sugar when we are carrying out a similar activity or when we find ourselves in a similar environment in the future. So, for example, if there is a piece of cake on your desk when you arrive at work because it is a colleague's birthday, your brain will create triggers linking the sugar to your arrival at work. This means that when you arrive at work and sit down at your desk the following day, your brain will prompt you to look for sugar. The 'desire for something sweet' will suddenly pop into your head.

If you consume sugar in response to this trigger you will strengthen it - making it easier for your brain to prompt you to look for sugar when you arrive at work in future and harder for the conscious part of your brain to block this prompt. You may find that you quickly get into the habit of eating a sugary treat each morning when you arrive at work and sit down at your desk. So when we eat sugar in response to a craving, we are not only creating External Triggers that change the foods that we choose to eat, we are also creating External Triggers that change our eating patterns - long after the craving that originally produced them has gone. Each time sugar crosses our path by chance we create these triggers so, over time, more and more places, activities and times of day can trigger our desire for sugar. But once again, it is our cravings that push this process into overdrive because they appear 'randomly' throughout the day driving us to consume sugar in new places, at new times and when we are doing new things.

Even if we consume a food that is already on our Sugar Map in response to a craving, such as a favourite chocolate bar, we are still creating new External Triggers that will change our eating patterns if we are consuming the sugar in a new place, at a new time or when we are doing a new activity.

We can begin to eat more treats between meals – a sugary snack when we arrive at our desk each morning or a doughnut and a chocolate bar on our trips to the mall for example. This change in our eating patterns can have a dramatic effect because, as you were probably told as a child, eating between meals ruins your appetite.

Normally we eat because 'ghrelin', a hormone that is produced by cells in our stomach, begins to build up when our stomach is empty. As ghrelin increases, our feelings of hunger become more intense. We start by feeling 'peckish' and end up feeling 'ravenous'. But when we eat high sugar foods between meals, we can break the link between hunger and eating and we can begin to eat in response to our External and Internal Triggers instead.

We eat more between meals (in response to the prompts that are created by our activities, our environment or our cravings) but less (or sometimes nothing at all) at meal times because eating between meals stops the ghrelin in our stomach from building up enough to make us feel hungry. This can create an erratic pattern of eating that we call 'grazing' where we eat a series of snacks during the day in place of meals.

Ironically, the pattern of eating that is created by our cravings can lead to more cravings. As you may remember, we can stop our blood sugar from falling between meals by converting stored fuel back into glucose but we can't do this when our Sugar Rationing Programme is active because a high level of insulin locks fuel into our cells - so when we skip a meal or eat too little our blood sugar can drop and a craving can result. We can become 'hungry' for sugar but not much else because our blood sugar can fall faster than ghrelin can build up - so our cravings for sugar always appear before our feelings of hunger.

For example, if we begin the day with a sugary snack at our desk we can create a surge in our blood sugar that will result in a drop that can trigger a mid-morning craving for sugar. If we grab a sugary snack in response to this craving, we may then eat less at lunchtime because our blood sugar will still be high and the ghrelin in our stomach may not have had a chance to build up so we won't feel hungry. But if we eat little (or nothing) at lunch time, our blood sugar can fall again - creating another craving in the afternoon. And eating in response to this craving can mean that we don't feel hungry as evening approaches so we have another snack instead of a meal - only to find that our cravings reappear with a vengeance later in the evening.

We sometimes think that it is good to eat frequently because it 'balances our blood sugar' but you shouldn't need to eat to be able to do this. If you feel tired, anxious or irritable when you don't eat, it's because your body is struggling to burn stored fuel - hunger is the only thing you should feel when you don't eat. As well as becoming more erratic, our eating patterns can also reverse.

Our Eating Pattern Can Reverse

Instead of eating most of our food during the day when we are active, we can begin to eat less in the morning and more in the evening. We eat too little during the day and too much late in the day - reversing the idea of breakfasting like a King, lunching like a Prince and dining like a pauper.

We Eat Less In The Morning

We may eat less in the morning because our blood sugar level can be unusually high at this time. This can happen because we release stored fuel during the night to stop our blood sugar from falling whilst we sleep (remember we use stress hormones to boost our blood sugar if the fuel that we have stored is locked into our cells) but if our cells are resistant to insulin, the glucose that we release can remain trapped in our bloodstream because our cells are reluctant to burn it. This means that our blood sugar can be high when we wake.[56] (High morning blood sugar is used as a test for insulin resistance).

When our blood sugar is high, we don't feel hungry so many of us skip breakfast and wait until our blood sugar drops before eating later in the day.

We Eat More In The Evening

If we eat little during the day our appetite may catch up with us later in the evening. It is thought that this can happen because when we eat in response to drops in our blood sugar and not to hunger and we begin to snack throughout the day, we may not eat enough to switch off

---

56   No appetite or nausea at breakfast is a symptom of adrenal hormones being activated at night, as is night waking. Kharrazian, *Brain*, p80

the ghrelin production in our stomach.[57] If ghrelin builds up during the day our appetite can appear at the end of the day instead of at the beginning.[58]

When this happens we may find ourselves raiding the cupboards for sugar in the evening because our appetite is at its highest when our willpower is at its lowest.

Evening Sugar Binge = High Appetite + Low Willpower

As you may remember, the conscious part of our brain has a limited 'tank' of fuel that it has to use to carry out all its functions - thinking, decision-making and planning for example – as well as blocking the prompts from our unconscious. By the end of the day we have less fuel available to block these prompts because much of it has been used to fuel our other activities.

Our sugar programmes are sent into overdrive by refined sugars because they create surges in our blood sugar and neurotransmitters that simply aren't supposed to be there. Our Sugar Seeking Programme tracks these High and Fast sugars because the surges that they create make them look like better sources of fuel than the Slow and Low ones that we are supposed to eat. But, as we've seen,

---

57   People who skip breakfast eat more during the day in part because ghrelin rises to high levels. Lustig, *Fat Chance*, p143
58   Fructose does not suppress ghrelin. Ibid p128

the high level of fructose and fast-digesting glucose that they contain can trigger our Sugar Rationing Programme.

When this programme becomes active, our attraction to sugar goes up but our ability to control the surges in our blood sugar goes down because we switch from burning fuel to storing it. When our cells become more reluctant to let glucose inside, we release more insulin to force them to respond. This can turn the surges in our blood sugar into drops and create the cravings that we struggle to resist.

Once we begin to consume sugar in response to our cravings, our sugar consumption can spiral out of control because every time we fail to block a craving, we create External Triggers that make lasting changes to our diet and eating patterns - prompting us to eat an increasing number of high sugar foods and to eat more erratically. This creates a vicious circle because as our diet is pulled further off course, the number of highs and lows in our blood sugar increases and this increases our cravings even further. The more cravings we have, the more sugar we consume because the conscious part of our brain won't have enough fuel to be able to block them all. And every time we consume sugar in response to a craving we expand our Sugar Map - giving the unconscious part of our brain more opportunities to spot sugar.

Our sugar consumption climbs because the unconscious

part of our brain prompts us to consume sugar over and over again, day after day, in response to all the External Triggers that it can see and all the Internal Triggers that our dietary habits create.

The more sugar we consume, the more visceral fat and insulin we produce which keeps our Sugar Rationing Programme active and our appetite for sugar permanently high. And our appetite for sugar increases even more[59] when we are busy, tired or stressed - perhaps because we are using up more of the fuel that our brain needs to be able to block the prompts from our unconscious on other things, perhaps because our brain increases its prompts for sugar to boost our feel-good neurotransmitters so that we feel better.[60]

The prompts from our brain are not easy to block because we haven't evolved to resist sugar, we have evolved to consume it - especially when our Sugar Rationing Programme is active and our brain thinks that our fuel stores are running low.

We don't notice the slow creep of sugar into our diet nor the constant tiny changes that it makes to our eating patterns because our diet is a collection of habits that are controlled by the unconscious part of our brain - which

59   Lack of sleep increases also ghrelin and reduces leptin. Gundry, *Diet Evolution*, p119
60   Ibid, p21

means that we are not aware of them. Unless there is a special reason for it to stand out in your mind, you will probably find it hard to remember what you ate on this day last week. You may even struggle to remember what you ate yesterday. The foods that we eat and the eating patterns that we follow can change enormously without us noticing. And because we associate sugar with a sweet taste, we don't think of an increase in starchy carbohydrates - such as bread, rice, pasta, or potatoes - as an increase in sugar. Just as we don't usually notice an increase in the number of savoury foods that we eat that contain 'hidden' sugars - such as the sauces that we use for cooking.

However, although we may not notice the impact that our cravings are having on our dietary habits, we do notice the increase in cravings that these habits produce. We don't like cravings so when they begin to interrupt our day more and more frequently we try to regain control.

Unfortunately, when we do this, we often increase our sugar consumption even more.

*

Why Trying To Control Our Cravings Makes Them Worse

Our cravings are hard to resist because the conscious part of our brain lacks the fuel that it needs to be able to block the prompts from our unconscious but many of us discover two things that seem to help – skipping meals and using stimulants.

Although skipping meals increases our cravings in the long term because it creates erratic eating patterns, in the short term it can appear to reduce them. This may be because our cravings drive us towards foods that create surges in our blood sugar that can lead to drops so eating less of these foods creates fewer drops and fewer cravings. This may particularly apply to breakfast.

We often begin to skip breakfast (if we haven't stopped eating it already) because eating it seems to make our cravings worse. Remember our cells are more resistant to insulin in the morning, thanks to the effect of cortisol, so surges in our blood sugar are more dramatic at this time. And a more dramatic surge can lead to a more dramatic drop that kicks off our sugar cravings. We sometimes find that we can push the first craving of the day back a little by cutting out breakfast.

We may also eat less at lunchtime because we find that eating lunch makes us feel sleepy. There is a natural drop in our energy level in the afternoon. Speakers and trainers call the post-lunch session the 'graveyard slot' because this is the time when the audience is the least responsive. So if we eat a lunch that creates a surge in our blood sugar, we can flood our brain with serotonin (which makes us feel relaxed) at the time when our energy levels are falling naturally. It's not a good sign if eating triggers your cravings or makes you feel either sleepy or energised. Eating should just take away your feelings of hunger[61].

Of course skipping meals doesn't get rid of our cravings it only delays them because, even though we may not be creating surges in our blood sugar, unless we eat our blood sugar will begin to drop anyway. But we may try to suppress them when they appear by using stimulants to boost our blood sugar and neurotransmitters - although we don't realise that this is what we are doing. We use caffeine, nicotine or alcohol (which is both a stimulant and a depressant) to lift our mood and suppress our cravings.[62]

We are often happy to skip meals and to rely on stimulants because we think that, if we eat small amounts during the day (and sometimes not at all), we will be able to 'balance out' all the extra sugar that we are eating as a result of our cravings and that this will enable us to lose

61   Kharrazian, *Brain*, p63
62   Kharrazian, *Brain*, p62, 74

any extra fat that we have stored. But of course, the fat remains because the sugary snacks that we are eating keep our insulin level high and our Sugar Rationing Programme switched on - preventing our fat stores from being burned.

And we will always give in to our cravings in the end - however hard we try - because we can't block all the prompts from our unconscious. We **can** control our cravings, but we can **never** control them for long. Sometimes we can be 'good' all day only to find that we eat our own body weight in sugar in the evening when we are tired. Sometimes we can be 'good' for a few days and then have a sudden binge when we feel stressed. And we can often unwittingly make things even worse because by trying to make up for our binges by cutting back on the amount that we eat the following day - which means that we skip more meals and use more stimulants.

Trying to keep our sugar consumption under control becomes an ongoing battle - and it is one that we are guaranteed to lose because the conscious part of our brain isn't always in control. When sugar becomes more of a torment than a treat, we vow to cut it out of our diet completely. But it is when we try to quit sugar that we realise just how little control we have over it.

In the next chapter, we'll look at what happens when we try to quit and we'll find out why it is so hard to do.

5

Why Sugar Is Hard To Quit

We may love sugar but we hate the cravings that it creates. It becomes increasingly difficult to think of sugar as a 'treat' when we are driven to leave the comfort of our sofa to head out into the rain to get it. When we spend more of our time craving sugar than we do enjoying it, we vow to cut it out of our diet. In this chapter, we'll look at why we choose to quit sugar in the ways that we do – by trying to remove it from our diet completely, by trying to cut back on the amount that we consume or by trying to find a suitable substitute - and we'll discover the reason why these attempts to control our cravings can lead to a lifelong battle with sugar.

How We Try To Regain Control

We are not aware of the workings of our body, nor of our Sugar Programmes. We don't know the amount of glucose in our bloodstream, nor the amount of each neurotransmitter in our brain. We don't know how resistant our cells are to insulin, nor how well the leptin signal is reaching our brain. And we are not aware of the External Triggers that make up our Sugar Map and create our dietary habits.

We are not aware of any of these things because they are all controlled by the unconscious part of our brain so when we want to get our sugar consumption under control, these aren't the things that we try to change. We focus instead on the only thing that we are aware of - our cravings.

But being aware of our cravings is not the same as being able to control them. We set ourselves up for failure right from the start because everything that we do to try to regain control is based on the mistaken belief that we **choose** to consume sugar in response to a craving. Since we are able to resist some of our cravings, some of the time, we believe that the conscious part of our brain is in control so we feel sure that we will be able to resist all of our cravings all of the time, once we have decided not to act on them. However, we soon find that resisting our cravings is not as easy as we expect it to be. Let's look at what happens when we try to quit sugar.

What Happens When We Quit Sugar

We usually quit sugar without any preparation because we think that all we need to do is to make the decision not to consume it. We simply choose a day to begin and vow that no more sugar will pass our lips from this moment onwards. Mondays are always popular because we like to make sure that we don't miss out on any sweet treats that may be on offer over the weekend. We may be about to quit sugar forever but we still want to enjoy it while we can. We avoid trying to quit before holidays too for the same reason. In fact, we often consume more sugar in the days before we quit because we like to consume all our favourite treats for the 'last time'.

Once we reach our chosen start date, we measure our success by counting the hours that have passed since we consumed our last sweet treat. We don't usually need to count for very long though because most of our attempts to quit are very short lived. Despite our initial confidence, we can often find ourselves consuming sugar again before the day is over because as soon as we quit sugar we lose our ability to resist it. This happens because we fall into the 'Willpower Trap'.

The Willpower Trap

When we give in to a craving we think that we have chosen to return to sugar because we value the pleasure that we get from our treats more than we value the satisfaction that we will feel when we get our sugar consumption under control. We call the ability to give up an immediate reward in order to gain a future reward 'willpower', so when we fail to resist our cravings, we think that we lack willpower.

We find this lack of willpower confusing because we really do hate our cravings and we really do feel committed to giving up sugar so we don't understand why we keep making the 'wrong decision'. We think that our inability to resist our cravings shows that we aren't as committed to our goal as we thought we were. However, if we could see the full picture, we would realise that our willpower isn't what we think it is.

Willpower isn't a measure of our commitment to quitting sugar, it's a measure of our ability to do so.[63] We think that willpower is the action of choosing a long-term reward over a short term one. But willpower is actually the action of using the conscious part of our brain to block a prompt from the unconscious part of our brain so that we stop ourselves from automatically responding to a

---

63   Self-control weakens as glucose levels fall. Lewis, *Impulse*

trigger. Our willpower doesn't depend on our motivation nor on our commitment, it simply depends on whether the conscious part of our brain has enough fuel to be able to block this prompt.

Because our commitment to quitting sugar and our ability to do so are not connected we can be totally committed to our goal and still find ourselves scoffing something sweet as fast as humanly possible. When our blood sugar and neurotransmitters are at a normal level and the conscious part of our brain has enough fuel to be able to block the prompts from our unconscious, sugar is easy to resist. We say that our willpower is high.

Normal Blood Sugar/ = Can Block → We Can Resist Neurotransmitters   Triggers   Sugar

High Willpower

But when our blood sugar and neurotransmitters drop and the conscious part of our brain lacks the fuel that it needs to block the prompts from our unconscious, sugar becomes much harder to resist. We say that our willpower is low.

Low Blood Sugar/ = Can't Block → We Can't Resist Neurotransmitters   Triggers   Sugar

Low Willpower

We expect our willpower to be constant but it's not. It varies throughout the day as our blood sugar and neurotransmitters rise and fall. When the conscious part of our brain has enough fuel to block a prompt from our unconscious, we can resist sugar and when it hasn't, we can't which is why we can resist some of our cravings some of the time but we can never resist all of our cravings all of the time.

And as we've seen, the Internal Triggers that create our cravings are always harder to block than the External Triggers that create our habits because our External Triggers are activated by things in the world around us but our cravings are activated by drops in our blood sugar and neurotransmitters - so they appear at the very time when our brain lacks fuel and our willpower is low. Our cravings feel as though they are out of control because they often are out of our (conscious) control.

When we quit, our cravings become even harder to resist because when we remove the sugar from our diet, we are also removing the fuel that the conscious part of our brain needs to be able to take action. We use up fuel every time we block a prompt from our unconscious so the very act of resisting a craving decreases our chances of resisting the next one.[64]

Dopamine, in particular, seems to be needed by the

64   Gaillot Matthew 2007, cited in Lewis, *Impulse*

conscious part of our brain to enable us to block the prompts from our unconscious so when we stop using sugar to boost our neurotransmitters and the amount of dopamine in our brain drops, our willpower disappears[65] and we quickly find ourselves returning to sugar. The more willpower we need, the less we have. We quit because our cravings feel out of control only to find that we have even less control over them than before.

The problem is that as soon as we add sugar back to our diet, the fuel supply to our brain is restored, so our willpower returns because the conscious part of our brain has the fuel that it needs to resist our cravings once again. This catches us in a trap because when our willpower is high we don't just feel confident about our ability to resist our cravings at that particular moment, we think that we will be able to resist our future cravings too. This happens because our brain creates our expectations of the future based on our experience of the present.[66]

So even though we may have just tried and failed to quit – often spectacularly - we are confident that our next attempt to quit will succeed. But of course, it never does because as soon as we switch off the supply of sugar again, we switch off our supply of Willpower.

---

65   Ibid
66   Unconscious brain determines expectation of the future. Kahneman, *Thinking*, Ch6

Our willpower always disappears when the sugar disappears and returns when the sugar returns - along with our certainty of success.[67]

Willpower High → We Think We Can Resist Sugar → We Quit → Our Willpower Disappears → We Return To Sugar → Our Willpower Returns

The belief that we can succeed, if just we try a little harder, turns the battle with our cravings into a lifelong war because it encourages us to keep trying to quit in the same way over and over again. We give up and our willpower disappears, we give in and our willpower returns. We always start out with great expectations and are always surprised when we fail because we are always sure that success is within our grasp.

Over time, we become increasingly frustrated by our lack of success because we think that we are choosing to return to sugar. We know that we **can** resist our cravings so we are confused about why we keep choosing to give in to them. At this point, we give ourselves a stern talking to. We really **do** want to quit. We really **are** committed. We really **will** try harder.

---

67   Ibid Ch 19 We cannot construct past states of knowledge or beliefs. We lose the ability to recall what we used to believe before our mind changed.

We can never succeed though because, if we do manage to resist our cravings for any length of time, we fall straight into the second trap – we plunge into Withdrawal.

The Withdrawal Trap

The more cravings we manage to resist, the worse we feel because we are removing the fuel that our brain needs to function. If we stop using sugar to boost our blood sugar, we need to release stress hormones to prop it up. And if we stop using sugar to boost our neurotransmitters, we are no longer releasing enough neurotransmitters to hit the reduced number of receptors in our brain. When we take away the fuel that our brain has come to depend on we become anxious, irritable and unable to focus.[68] We call the period of fatigue, low mood and general misery that results, 'Withdrawal'. Not only do we feel bad, our cravings become more intense because our brain is trying to drive us back to sugar so that it has the fuel that it needs.

We are always surprised by this increase in our cravings because we don't realise that we have become dependent on sugar. We think we are 'missing' the pleasure that we got from our treats more than we expected that we would. But, in reality, our cravings have increased because our brain

68   Kharrazian, *Brain*, p59-62

is 'missing' the fuel that it needs to function. (Once again, it's a lack of dopamine that has been linked with the dramatic increase in our cravings[69]).

When we remove sugar from our diet, we are not just removing the cause of the drops in our blood sugar and neurotransmitters, we are also removing the thing that fixes them - at least temporarily. We plunge into Withdrawal because we are withdrawing the fuel that our brain needs. Trying to take control of sugar by resisting our cravings is not just unpleasant, it's ineffective because, when our brain needs sugar to function, taking that sugar away will only ever make our cravings worse.

The 'Withdrawal Trap' spells the end of most of our attempts to quit. In fact, if we make it as far as Withdrawal we are often just prolonging the agony before we return to sugar. We quit to escape our cravings, but we are forced back to sugar again because they grow worse. And when we return to sugar, we often do it in style.

We often work our way through our favourite treats all over again - even though we were sure when we ate them just a few days ago that we were eating them for the last time. We think that if we fail to stick to our promise to quit by eating a piece of cake, we can't 'fail more' by eating two pieces of cake or even two whole cakes. This sugar binge is so common that there is actually a name for it

---

69   Lustig, *Fat Chance*, p54

– the 'What The Hell' effect. We think that this binge happens because we have missed our treats so much. But we actually binge when we return to sugar because the reward that we get for consuming sugar increases even more when we quit.

As you may remember from Chapter 3, our leptin level drops as soon as our fuel supply drops so that our appetite is increased to protect our fat stores. Sugar is a very concentrated fuel so when we quit sugar, we are cutting our fuel supply and decreasing our leptin level. Remember, the leptin signal to our brain is already being blocked by the insulin that we are releasing in response to glucose. So when we quit sugar we have a blocked leptin signal **and** less leptin so the reward that we get from sugar increases even more. Sugar becomes more attractive and we can eat more of it which means that when we give in to a craving after we've quit we consume a lot more sugar - creating the 'What The Hell' effect that leads to a binge.

We feel better once we have consumed sugar again because our blood sugar and neurotransmitters get a big boost so we escape the unpleasantness of Withdrawal. But the relief that we feel when we get our treats back doesn't last long because our cravings quickly reappear. Our willpower returns too so we begin to feel annoyed that we returned to sugar so quickly. We feel sure that we will be able to resist our cravings on our next attempt – if we can just try a little harder. We tell ourselves that we were just too busy, too tired or too stressed to succeed the last time we tried to quit. So we pick another date (usually after we've had time to consume all our favourite treats 'for the last time' once again and we've got the weekend out of the way and our holiday and that birthday night out) and then we try to quit sugar in the same way all over again.

Unfortunately, we get the same results all over again too.

*

Sugar is hard to quit because we are trying to use the conscious part of our brain to stop our brain from getting the fuel that it needs. Every time we cut the sugar from our diet our cravings increase, we feel bad and our willpower disappears because once we begin consuming sugar, our brain struggles to function without it.

We find that we are forced back to sugar again and again - however hard we try - because we are taking away the fuel that we need to resist it. So despite all our efforts, our sugar consumption remains unchanged. In fact, we may even consume more sugar than usual by having a 'Last Time' sugar binge at the beginning of an attempt to quit and a 'What the Hell' sugar binge at the end – especially if we are trying to quit on a weekly basis.

However, because we don't realise that our brain is driving us back to sugar to get the fuel that it needs, we think that we are failing to stick to our vow to quit because we just can't live without our treats. When we think that we are too weak-willed to be able to cut sugar out of our diet completely, we try to work around our lack of willpower by choosing an easier goal.

Instead of trying to remove all the sugar from our diet we decide that we will just try to 'cut back' on it. We think that resisting some of our cravings, some of the time will be easier than trying to resist all of our cravings, all of the time. But cutting back on sugar isn't the easier option that it appears to be.

Let's look at what happens when we try to lower our sugar consumption, instead of trying to quit sugar completely.

*

Why Cutting Back On Sugar Doesn't Work

We expect cutting back to be easier than quitting because we think that we won't miss sugar quite so much if we have an occasional treat to look forward to. We hope that by keeping some of our treats we will avoid the increase in cravings and decrease in willpower that happens whenever we quit.

But of course, we don't because, when we need sugar to prop up our blood sugar and neurotransmitters, any reduction in sugar makes our cravings worse. The more fuel we take away, the worse our cravings become and the worse we feel. And the promise of a treat does nothing to improve our ability to resist our cravings because we are still removing the fuel that the conscious part of our brain needs to be able to take action. The more fuel we take away, the lower our willpower becomes.

We usually manage to avoid going into Withdrawal when we cut back but only because we find an excuse to give in to a craving before our neurotransmitters fall too far. Instead of the 'one strike and we're out policy' that we have when we try to quit completely, we are able to give in to our cravings without thinking that we are 'back at the beginning'.

This means that we can disguise our failure to be able to block a craving simply by finding a reason to justify our 'decision' to consume sugar. So when we are unable to resist a craving, we simply think of a reason to explain why we 'deserved' the treat.

We can find endless excuses, "It's the weekend", "I've had a hard day" or "I've finished my report", for example. It's a type of 'Halo Effect'. If we can find a 'good' reason to explain our 'bad' behaviour we don't feel that our cravings are out of control. We feel better when we think that we are consuming sugar because it's a special occasion and not just something that we are powerless to stop.

Even successfully resisting our cravings gives us an excuse to indulge - the "I've been 'good' all day so I deserve a treat" excuse. We fail to see the irony when we 'celebrate' resisting sugar by consuming it.

Cutting back has little impact on our sugar consumption because, although we think that we are choosing to treat ourselves, in reality we are simply finding a reason to excuse our behaviour whenever we fail to stop ourselves from responding to a prompt from our brain. We can't cut much sugar out of our diet anyway before the drop in our fuel supply pushes us into Withdrawal and increases our cravings. As we've seen, every time we successfully resist a craving our brain has less fuel so we increase our need for sugar and reduce our willpower.

Eventually, cutting back begins to feel too much like hard work because, whether we were aiming to consume sugar once a day or once a week, only after the gym or only at the weekend, we are always unable to stick to the limits that we set for ourselves and we are constantly forced to move the goalposts. When we find that we don't even have enough willpower to manage to cut back we begin to look for an easier solution – one that means that we don't have to give up our treats at all.

Since we are obviously too weak-willed to resist sugar, we decide to find a sugar that we won't have to resist. We hope that by finding a 'healthy' sugar, we will be able to feel good about ourselves - no matter how much we consume. But unfortunately, like cutting back, using a sugar substitute is not the easy option that it appears to be.

Why Sugar Substitutes Don't Work

When we decide that we are too weak-willed to be able to cut back on sugar, we begin an (often frantic) search for 'healthy' sugar that we can use as a substitute. I call the search for a substitute the 'Brownie Factor' because what we want is a warm chocolate brownie that tastes just as good as the sugar-filled version but is magically made out of stuff that is good for us. Whilst we use the 'Halo Effect' to find a 'good' reason for our 'bad' behaviour, we use the Brownie Factor to try to make our 'bad' behaviour seem 'good'.

We are relieved to find that the internet is packed with recipes for 'sugar-free' brownies and other 'guilt-free' treats. (We particularly like brownies because cocoa contains stimulants which give us an extra boost).[70] We find a whole new world of sugars and we are sure that one of them will be right for us. Using a sugar substitute makes us feel better about our inability to quit or cut back because as long as we are avoiding white sugar, we think that we are being 'good'. We can have a diet that is packed with High & Fast sugars and still believe that we are sugar-free (I call this the 'No Sugar, Sugar Diet').

There are three types of sugar substitute that we use to replace the 'white sugar' in our diet:- fruit, 'natural' sugars and artificial sweeteners. We feel that we are being good when we consume fruit because it contains a lot of nutrients. We feel that we are being good when we consume refined sugars like agave, honey or maple syrup because we believe that they are more 'natural' than white sugar. And we can also feel that we are being good when we consume artificial sweeteners because, although they are not natural, they are calorie-free so we don't think that they count as sugar at all. The problem is that swapping to a sugar substitute won't do anything to stop our cravings. In fact, substitutes can often make our cravings worse. Let's find out why this can happen.

---

70   Kharrazian, Brain, p338

Sugar Substitutes Can Send Us Into Withdrawal

Often our first instinct is to try to swap refined sugar for the natural sugars that are found in fruit. Fruit is packed with nutrients so we feel that we are being 'good' when we consume it and we think that the sweet taste will satisfy our cravings for something sweet.

However, if we swap to fruit that contain Low & Slow sugars (such as berries), our cravings go up and our willpower goes down in the same way that they do when we quit sugar completely. We fall into the Willpower and Withdrawal Traps in exactly the same way because we are no longer creating the surges of glucose that we need to boost our blood sugar and neurotransmitters.

When our brain no longer has the fuel that it needs we are driven back to sugar so pretty soon the only berries in our diet are the blueberries in our muffin. Fruit is a healthy food but it doesn't help us to get rid of our cravings for sugar.

Once we realise that swapping to low-sugar fruits makes our cravings worse, we often swap to high-sugar fruits, such as dates, or to other refined sugars that we think are 'natural'. These substitutes **can** satisfy our cravings and keep us out of Withdrawal but only because they behave in exactly the same way as the refined sugar that we are trying so hard to avoid.

Sugar Substitutes Can Disrupt Our Blood Sugar

All 'Slow and Low' sugars become 'High and Fast' when they are removed from their original source - even the 'natural' ones - so these sugars create surges in our blood sugar in the same way that sugar does. And dates, which are another popular choice, are one of the few natural foods that also create these surges. In fact, dates contain so much fast-digesting glucose that they are even higher on the glycemic index than white sugar.

Foods that contain artificial sweeteners can also disrupt our blood sugar – even though they don't contain any glucose. This can happen for two reasons. Firstly, because the food itself may be high in fast-digesting glucose – even if it isn't in the sweetener. An artificially sweetened muffin will still be high on the glycemic index because it contains flour which ranks higher on the scale than sugar. Secondly, although we may not think that sweeteners count as sugar, our brain thinks that they do. When we consume a food with a sweet taste, our brain is fooled into thinking that we have found sugar so it tells our pancreas to release insulin to move the glucose that it is expecting out of our bloodstream and into our cells. This can result in a drop in our blood sugar because some of the existing glucose is removed – so even if we don't create a surge in our blood sugar, we can still create a drop.[71]

---

71   Hyman, Mark. *The Blood Sugar Solution 10-Day Detox Diet, p36*

Sugar Substitutes Can Disrupt Our Neurotransmitters

Sugar substitutes can disrupt our neurotransmitters too. Our brain rewards us when we consume dates and 'natural' refined sugars because it thinks that they are great sources of fuel but they create surges in our neurotransmitters in the same way that sugar does because they are so concentrated. Artificial sweeteners also create a feel-good reward in our brain because, even though they are calorie free, the sweet taste fools our brain into thinking that we have found fuel.

We wouldn't bother to use these substitutes in place of sugar if they didn't create surges in our neurotransmitters because they wouldn't make us feel good and they wouldn't satisfy our cravings. The problem is that our brain protects itself from the surges in our neurotransmitters that we get from artificial sweeteners and other refined sugars by switching off the receptors on our neurons - just as it does when we consume 'white' sugar.[72]

Our cravings simply continue if we swap to these sugars and if we stop consuming them, our neurotransmitters drop and we go into Withdrawal in exactly the same way as we do when we remove white sugar from our diet. We might think that we have quit sugar, but our brain disagrees.

---

72   Lustig, *Fat Chance*, p194

Sugar Substitutes Can Activate Our Sugar Programmes

Sugar substitutes activate our Sugar Seeking Programme just like 'regular' sugar because all foods that create a reward in our brain create External Triggers. Everything with a sweet taste is added to our Sugar Map because our brain doesn't distinguish between different types of sugar. It tracks these sugars - and prompts us to consume them – in the same way as sugar. These sugars can also activate our Sugar Rationing Programme.

If the substitutes that we choose contain fast-digesting glucose and/or fructose they continue to create the Feast and Famine triggers (visceral fat and insulin) that trigger this programme. And perhaps surprisingly, artificial sweeteners can activate this Programme too – despite containing neither glucose nor fructose. In fact, studies suggest that artificial sweeteners may switch off the insulin receptors on our cells even faster than sugar. For example, rats that were fed artificially sweetened food ate more food and gained 14% more body fat in just 2 weeks – even if they ate fewer calories – than rats whose food was sweetened with sugar.[73]

There are two possible reasons for this. If our brain thinks that we have found sugar and we release insulin in response, the insulin can block the leptin signal to our brain - so artificial sweeteners may still create the Famine

---

[73]   Hyman, *Blood Sugar,* p36

signal because they can hide our fat stores from our brain. But these sweeteners may also trigger insulin resistance by changing the proportions of 'good' and 'bad' bacteria that live in our gut.

Just like fructose, artificial sweeteners feed our bad bacteria allowing them to reproduce quickly and to crowd out our good bacteria.[74] One study showed that Splenda reduced good bacteria by 50%.[75] These bad bacteria may then release substances into our bloodstream that can switch off the insulin receptors on our cells. (Our gut bacteria are also involved in the manufacture of dopamine)[76].

The extra effort that we make to stick to substitutes and to 'avoid' sugar is wasted because when we swap to a substitute – even an artificial one - we aren't removing the sugar from our diet at all. And we are not reducing our dependency on it. Sugar substitutes don't reduce our cravings because they continue to disrupt our blood sugar and neurotransmitters and they don't reduce our desire for sugar either because we create External Triggers when we consume them.

---

74   Lustig, *Fat Chance*, p194

75   Abou-Donia, Mohamed B. et al. "Splenda Alters Gut Microflora And Increases Intestinal P-Glycoprotein And Cytochrome P-450 In Male Rats". Journal of Toxicology and Environmental Health, Part A 71.21 (2008): 1415-1429 cited in Gedgaudas, *Primal Body*, p175

76   Kharrazian, *Brain*, p346

Sugar substitutes of any type, in large or small amounts, can't fix the problem that sugar has created. But we like to use them because when we swap to using a substitute, we think that we are avoiding sugar so we feel better about our inability to resist our cravings.

The final problem is that swapping to a sugar substitute makes our life harder because these sugars aren't as easy to find as white sugar. Often, the only way to ensure that we stick with our chosen substitute is to make our own treats and to carry them with us at all times. We may be happy to do this at the start of our 'sugar-free' diet - when we are brimming with enthusiasm - but it is hard to keep this up for months or years on end. We usually end up drifting back to sugar again because, when our brain prompts us to search for sugar it doesn't care what type of sugar we find, so when our chosen substitute isn't available we simply grab the regular stuff.

*

The path that most of us follow is to begin by trying to remove all the sugar from our diet. But once we find out that this is unpleasant (because we plunge into Withdrawal) and impossible to do (because our willpower disappears), we try to cut back instead. Cutting back removes less sugar so it's less unpleasant (because we can avoid Withdrawal) and it's not as hard to do (because we can use the Halo Effect to excuse any lapses in our willpower). But cutting back on sugar doesn't have any impact on our cravings at all – except to make them worse if we try to cut too much sugar out of our diet. And it has little impact on our sugar consumption because we still consume sugar whenever we lack the fuel that we need to block the prompt from our unconscious. So eventually we stop trying to reduce the amount of sugar in our diet and we try to find a 'healthy' sugar instead.

Quit	→ We Cut Out Our Treats	→ Our Cravings Increase Dramatically
Cut Back	→ We Cut Out Some Treats	→ Our Cravings Grow Worse
Substitute	→ We Keep Our Treats	→ We Keep Our Cravings

Each strategy is easier to carry out than the last but only because each one has **less impact** on our sugar consumption than the last. When we begin to search for sugar substitutes, we are accepting that we have lost the battle against our cravings. We are no longer trying to get rid of them, we are just trying to find the best way to live with them.

Sugar is hard to quit because the more sugar we remove from our diet, the more our cravings increase and the lower our willpower becomes so we are forced back to sugar over and over again. Of course, as we've seen, our biology is against us because we haven't evolved to resist sugar, we've evolved to consume as much of it as possible.

But if we are programmed to seek it out, we have easy access to it all year round and it makes massive changes to our body and brain that keep us hooked, can we ever escape? Is there an easy way to get rid of our cravings?

Fortunately, the answer is 'yes'. So now that you understand why quitting, cutting back or using a substitute will only ever make your cravings worse, it's time to find out how to reverse the changes that sugar has made so that you can get rid of your cravings and get your sugar consumption under control.

The second book in this series, 'The Easy Way To Quit Sugar' will explain how to do this.

The Easy Way To Quit Sugar

The Easy Way To Quit Sugar explains how you can get rid of your cravings by doing the opposite of what you are doing now – by removing your brain's need for sugar, instead of trying to remove the sugar that your brain needs. The good news is that you can do this by making just two key changes to your diet. You can make these changes easily whether you are a vegan, a veggie or an omnivore. There are no recipes to learn, no meal plans to follow and no new ingredients to hunt down.

And once you have regained control, you will be able to stay in control so that you can add sugar back to your diet without worrying that your cravings will return in the future.

Before you begin to take action don't forget to download your free guide to measuring the effects of sugar on your body which you can find at the following address:-

http://www.janeneish.com/measure/

One last thing.... If you enjoyed this book I'd be very grateful if you'd post a short review on Amazon to let me know what you liked and what you found most useful. I read all the reviews and your support really **does** make a difference. To leave a review simply visit this book's Amazon page and scroll down to the find the button that says 'Write A Customer Review'. You should be able to go straight to the page if you type the following address into your browser:-

http://viewbook.at/hardtoquit/

Thank you!

Suggested Reading

Skinny Chicks Don't Eat Salad – Christine Avanti

The Plant Plus Solution – Joan Borysenko

The De Vany Diet – Arthur De Vany

The Power Of Habit – Charles Duhigg

Primal Body, Primal Mind – Nora T. Gedgaudas

Dr Gundry's Diet Evolution – Steven R Gundry

10 Day Detox Diet – Dr Mark Hyman

Thinking Fast & Slow – Daniel Kahneman

Why Isn't My Brain Working – Datis Kharrazion

Impulse – Dr David Lewis

Fat Chance. The Bitter Truth About Sugar – Dr Robert Lustig

The Procrastination Equation – Dr Piers Steel

Good Calories, Bad Calories - Gary Taubes

Acknowledgements

They say that writing a book is an act of insanity and it certainly felt like that at times - especially as I started writing this book at the beginning of what turned out to be a very turbulent time in my life. You are holding a copy now only because I had a great team to help me. So I'd like to thank everyone who was part of the editorial team as well as the friends who continued to support me even when I became a terrible recluse.

Sara, Sue, Denise, Sarah, Ruth, Christine, Hazel, Maddy, Suzy, Elizabeth, Karen, Chiara, Sue, Maxine, Sandra, Mini, Sheila, Pat, Angie, Matt & Brendan – thank you all.

Special thanks to Emma, Dominique & Claire for going above and beyond the call of duty.

And of course, a huge thank you to John who suffered more than anyone during the production of this book.

You all did such a great job that I'm going to do it all over again!

Read on for details about Jane's next book.

The Easy Way To
QUIT SUGAR

Stop Your Sugar Cravings, Boost Your
Willpower & Discover The Sugar Free
Diet That Is Right For You

JANE NEISH

The Easy Way To Quit Sugar

Stop waging war on sugar and discover the secrets that will free you from your cravings forever.

If you take away your brain's need for sugar you will have no problem controlling your sugar consumption. The **Easy Way To Quit Sugar** reveals how you can get back in control and stay in control by reversing the changes that sugar has made to your body and brain that are keeping you hooked.

- You can switch off your cravings **and** the urge that you have to consume sugar whenever it crosses your path simply by making just two simple changes to your diet.
- You don't need to follow a new diet, learn new recipes or hunt down new ingredients.
- You don't need to use willpower to battle against your cravings, you don't need to use sugar substitutes and you don't need to go through Withdrawal. This really is the easy way to quit.

And once you're back in control, you will be able to keep sugar out of your diet without feeling deprived or add sugar back to your diet without seeing the return of your cravings.

Jane Neish worked in television before completing a Master's degree in Employment Analysis and setting up a business as a corporate trainer and executive coach. A lifelong sugar addict, she was struck by the fact that many of her clients were struggling with sugar cravings and she began to look for ways to help them – and herself. She discovered that controlling your sugar cravings is impossible but that switching them off is not. This discovery changed Jane's life - and her business - eventually leading to the 'Switch Off Your Sugar Cravings' programme that she teaches today.

Jane now works as a specialist 'Sugar Coach' – running a private practice in Manchester and delivering workshops throughout the UK. Her first book, 'Why It's Hard To Quit Sugar', has sold in 13 countries, reaching No.1 in the Amazon bestseller charts in the UK and No.2 in the US. She is currently finishing a second book – The Easy Way To Quit Sugar - and developing an online coaching program. Jane lives in Cheshire. She had a full social life and many hobbies until she made the decision to begin writing books.

To find out how to switch off your sugar cravings visit
www.janeneish.com.

www.ingramcontent.com/pod-product-compliance
Lightning Source LLC
Chambersburg PA
CBHW062206280526
45788CB00001B/462